The COMPLETE GUIDE to CARB COUNTING 3rd Edition

How to take the mystery out of carb counting and improve your blood glucose control

by

Hope S. Warshaw,
MMSc, RD, CDE, BC-ADM

Karmeen Kulkarni,
MS, RD, CDE, BC-ADM

 American Diabetes Association.

Director, Book Publishing, Abe Ogden; Acquisitions Editor, Victor Van Beuren; Editor, Greg Guthrie; Production Manager, Melissa Sprott; Composition, ADA; Cover Design, Vis-à-Vis Creative Concepts; Writer, Jennifer Arnold; Printer, Thomson-Shore, Inc..

Printed in the United States of America
1 3 5 7 9 10 8 6 4 2

The suggestions and information contained in this publication are generally consistent with the *Clinical Practice Recommendations* and other policies of the American Diabetes Association, but they do not represent the policy or position of the Association or any of its boards or committees. Reasonable steps have been taken to ensure the accuracy of the information presented. However, the American Diabetes Association cannot ensure the safety or efficacy of any product or service described in this publication. Individuals are advised to consult a physician or other appropriate health care professional before undertaking any diet or exercise program or taking any medication referred to in this publication. Professionals must use and apply their own professional judgment, experience, and training and should not rely solely on the information contained in this publication before prescribing any diet, exercise, or medication. The American Diabetes Association—its officers, directors, employees, volunteers, and members—assumes no responsibility or liability for personal or other injury, loss, or damage that may result from the suggestions or information in this publication.

⊗ The paper in this publication meets the requirements of the ANSI Standard Z39.48-1992 (permanence of paper).

ADA titles may be purchased for business or promotional use or for special sales. To purchase more than 50 copies of this book at a discount, or for custom editions of this book with your logo, contact the American Diabetes Association at the address below, at booksales@diabetes.org, or by calling 703-299-2046.

American Diabetes Association
1701 North Beauregard Street
Alexandria, Virginia 22311

DOI: 10.2337/ 9781580404365

Library of Congress Cataloging-in-Publication Data

Warshaw, Hope S., 1954-
  Complete guide to carb counting : how to take the mystery out of carb counting and improve your blood glucose control / Hope S. Warshaw, Karmeen Kulkarni. -- 3rd ed.
    p. cm.
  Includes bibliographical references and index.
  ISBN 978-1-58040-436-5 (pbk.)
  1. Diabetes--Diet therapy. 2. Food--Carbohydrate content. I. Kulkarni, Karmeen, 1953- II. Title.
  RC662.W313 2011
  616.4'620654--dc22

                                                    2011000233

This book is dedicated to all people with diabetes.

We hope it provides you with the knowledge and skills to make
carb counting a central part of your diabetes care
and helps you to achieve the diabetes control and
quality of life that you desire.

◆ ◆

Foreword

Carbohydrates (or more precisely, lack thereof) have received a lot of attention over the last decade. It seems that with the recent popularity of low-carbohydrate diets on the market (diets, it should be noted, that have not been backed by serious scientific evidence), it's nearly impossible to visit a grocery store, eat at a restaurant, or even open a newspaper without hearing about carbs. For those with diabetes, attention to carbohydrate is nothing new. Even before the discovery of insulin, early meal planning techniques focused on restricting carbohydrate intake. Over time, our understanding of carbohydrates improved. As the decades passed and research continued, it became clear that carbohydrates had the largest impact on blood glucose levels. Eventually, it was shown that not only sugar had this effect, but all carbohydrates. By the turn of the century, one of the main challenges of diabetes therapy was to match carbohydrate content to insulin availability (whether made by your body or injected from outside).

Just from a conceptual point of view, this notion seems easy enough to understand. However, as anyone who has ever tried to put this theory into practice appreciates, the process can be exceedingly difficult. Immediately a host of questions springs to mind: What is a carbohydrate? What foods contain carbohydrate? How much carbohydrate should a person eat? How do you count all of this carbohydrate? And perhaps ultimately, how does this help with diabetes management? Suddenly, what at first seemed like a simple matter of adding numbers can become overwhelming.

Fortunately, this is a good time to be a "carb counter." There are a variety of resources available to help you in your pursuit of counting carbohydrates. Nutrition information detailing the amount of carbohydrate in foods is widely available, whether it is printed on the Nutrition Facts label on packaged food products, available in a menu at a restaurant, listed on a website, or catalogued in a carb count book. Many cookbooks, including all of those from the American Diabetes Association, list the nutrition information for their recipes. Scales and measuring devices, essential pieces of advanced carb counting, can be easily ordered from websites. In other words, the tools and aids available to you as a beginning carb counter are almost unlimited. Be sure to make these tools a part of your diabetes management. Recent studies have shown that the majority of people who count carbohydrate misestimate what they are actually eating. The reason for this, in my view, is not that the tools and aids are ineffective, but that they are not used effectively.

Furthermore, tools and aids can only do so much. They are not a method. Just because you have a hammer and saw doesn't mean you can build a house. To move forward you need a clear and cohesive blueprint. To build a strong carb counting program, think of this book as your blueprint. Within these pages, the internationally known authors provide a simple, easy-to-follow carb counting plan that can be tailored to any diabetes management regimen. They teach you how carbohydrate affects your blood glucose, how to use the tools available to you, why different sources of carbohydrate act differently in your body, and much more. They provide tips and tricks to make the process easier. And they present all of this information in a clear, easy-to-understand format that makes the process of learning as simple as possible.

Those who are new to carb counting often find that they have a lot of questions. However, all of these can be distilled down to two basic questions that form the foundation for the rest: Why should I count carbohydrates? And how do I count carbohydrates? The answers to both can be found in this book, which should be read by every physician, educator, and individual with diabetes. I teach our students that we never stop learning, no matter how much we think we know about a topic. It is for this reason that this most recent edition of *Complete Guide to Carb Counting* needs to be a part of every diabetes library, no matter if you are a health care professional or a person living with diabetes or both.

Irl B. Hirsch, MD
January 2011
Seattle, WA

Acknowledgments

We thank a number of colleagues who have provided valuable critiques on the three editions of *Complete Guide to Carb Counting*. These individuals include Sandy Gillespie, MMSc, RD, CDE; David Shade, MD; Anne Daly, MS, RD, CDE; Patti Geil, MS, RD, FADA, CDE; Joan Hill, RD, CDE, LD; Lea Ann Holzmeister, RD, CDE; and John White, PA, PharmD. We are also grateful to Irl Hirsch, MD, for writing the Foreword for the second and third editions of this book.

Thanks to the staff at ADA—Abe Ogden, Greg Guthrie, Jennifer Arnold, and Heschel Falek—who helped edit and prepare the manuscript for publication and developed marketing and publicity to ensure the success of this book.

I would also like to thank my family: Rajiv, my husband, and my daughter Anjali. Thanks go out to all of the people with diabetes with whom I have had the privilege to work, who taught me so much.

—*Karmeen Kulkarni*

1

◆ ◆

What Is Carb Counting?

Would you like to have a better sense of when your blood glucose is going to rise and be able to predict how high it might go today, tomorrow, or the next day? If your answer is YES, then carbohydrate counting—"carb counting" for short—might be an approach to planning your meals that works for you.

Carb counting is not a one-size-fits-all meal planning method. It is simply a method to help you plan and eat balanced meals and control your blood glucose level along with the other elements of your diabetes care plan, such as medications and exercise.

In This Chapter, You'll Learn:

Basic facts about carbohydrate

Which foods contain carbohydrate

How carbohydrate affects blood glucose

About the meal planning approach called carbohydrate counting

Why Count Carbs?

Foods contain varying amounts of carbohydrate, protein, fat, vitamins, minerals, and water. When you use carb counting, you focus on the carbohydrate in foods. Why is that? Because carbohydrate raises your blood glucose more—and more quickly—than the two other nutrients that provide calories—protein and fat (excluding alcohol).

1

Adding up the amount of carbohydrate in each meal and snack that you eat each day can help you keep your blood glucose at a steady level, adjust your insulin as needed (if you take it), and feel your best.

Variety: The Spice of Life

Carb counting also allows you to enjoy a wide variety of foods, as long as you eat about the same amount of carbohydrate at each meal and snack each day. The *foods* don't need to remain the same, but the *amount of carbohydrate* should. When you eat about the same amount of carbohydrate at each meal, day in and day out, your blood glucose levels are more likely to fall into a steady pattern. That means better blood glucose control for you.

Carb Counting May Not Be Right for Everyone

As you learn more about carb counting in the pages ahead, ask yourself whether you think this approach will fit your needs and lifestyle. In Chapter 2 you'll do a self-assessment to determine whether carb counting is right for you. There's another self-assessment in Chapter 11 to help you determine whether you want or need to progress from basic to advanced carb counting. We'll explain more as we go along—for now, it's time to learn which foods contain carbohydrate.

Which Foods Contain Carbohydrate?

Most people tend to equate carbohydrate with starches. Starches, such as potatoes, breads, and pasta, do contain carbohydrate, but they're not the only foods under the "carbohydrate umbrella." Here is a complete list of the food groups whose calories come mainly from carbohydrate:
  • Starches—bread, cereal, crackers, rice, and pasta
  • Starchy vegetables—peas, beans, lentils, potatoes, and corn
  • Fruit and fruit juice

- Nonstarchy vegetables—tomatoes, cauliflower, and carrots
- Dairy foods—milk, yogurt, and other dairy foods
- Sugary drinks—regular soda, fruit punch, sports drinks, and flavored waters
- Sweets—candy, cakes, cookies, and pies

After reading this list, you might wonder which foods do not contain carbohydrate. There are a few:

- meats (red meat, poultry, seafood, and eggs)
- fats (oil, butter, and nuts)

Although these foods that don't contain carbohydrate won't be part of your daily carb counting totals, you still need to pay attention to them. They contain calories and other nutrients that are also important to a healthy eating plan. You will learn more about protein and fats and how they affect eating plans in Chapter 4.

How Much Carbohydrate Is in These Foods?

The list of foods above includes general groups of foods that contain carbohydrate. But within each food group, there can be a wide range in the actual amount of carbohydrate in each food. For example, the amount of carbohydrate in dairy foods varies quite a bit. On average, 8 ounces of most cheeses contains about 8 grams of carbohydrate, whereas 8 ounces of milk contains 12 grams of carbohydrate.

You can see more examples of this in Table 1-1 on page 4, and in Appendix 1 at the back of the book. As you learn more, and start using carb counting in your meal planning, you'll rely on resources like these to help you determine the carb count in everything from apples to zucchini. For now, focus on the some common, simple foods and how they affect your blood glucose.

How Does Carb Counting Help with Blood Glucose Control?

Your blood glucose levels are related to the amount of carbohydrate you eat. If you regularly track the amount of carbohydrate

Table 1-1 Nutrients

Food group	Serving*	Carbohydrate (g)	Protein (g)	Fat (g)
Bread, white	1 slice (1 oz)	14.3	2.2	0.9
Corn flakes cereal, dry	3/4 cup	18.2	1.4	†
Pasta, cooked	1/3 cup	14.3	2.7	†
Baked potato w/ skin	1/4 (3 oz)	18.4	1.7	0.1
Peaches, fresh	1 large	15.5	1.4	0.5
Peaches, canned, no sugar added	1/2 cup	18.3	0.6	0
Broccoli, cooked	1/2 cup	5.6	1.9	0.3
Broccoli, raw	1 cup	6	2.6	0.4
Milk, fat-free	1 cup	12.3	8.7	0.7
Yogurt, plain, fat-free	2/3 cup	12.5	9.3	0.3
Brownie, unfrosted	1 oz	14.2	1.8	8.2
Ground beef, 95% lean	3 oz cooked	0	21.9	5
Margarine	1 tsp	0	0	3.8
Mayonnaise, regular	1 tsp	1.2	0	1.6

*Servings are from *Choose Your Foods: Exchange Lists for Meal Planning* published by ADA and The American Dietetic Association, 2008.
†Depends on the product.

you eat at a meal and check your blood glucose levels one to two hours after that meal, you'll hopefully detect patterns. That's what carb counting is all about. Monitoring the amount of carbohydrate you eat, and eating about the same amount at each meal, will help you keep your blood glucose levels on target throughout the day. This will help you feel your best and allow you to manage your blood glucose medication effectively.

In Chapter 3, we'll talk more about the data you need to record, how to record it, and how to use your results.

What's So Important about Controlling Blood Glucose Levels?

When you get and keep your blood glucose levels in your target ranges, you feel better. You also can help prevent and/or delay the complications of diabetes, such as heart, eye, and kidney problems. Think of blood glucose control like walking on a balance beam— you don't want to fall off on either side. There are dangers associated with both high blood glucose and low blood glucose (if you are on certain diabetes medications), so you want to stay right in the middle. Hypoglycemia is another word for low blood glucose. Hyperglycemia is another word for high blood glucose.

Table 1-2 gives you the target blood glucose levels that the American Diabetes Association (ADA) recommends. Ask your health care provider what your target levels should be; yours may be different from the ones in the table for a variety of reasons. For example, a pregnant woman may have lower target levels and an older person at risk for hypoglycemia may have higher target levels.

Table 1-2 Target Ranges for Blood Glucose and A1C Levels

Test	Goal
Average fasting and premeal blood glucose	70–130 mg/dl
Average postmeal blood glucose level (1–2 hours after the start of a meal)	<180 mg/dl
A1C (%)	<7% (normal range is based on 4–6%)

Basic Facts about Carbohydrate

When you eat any type of carbohydrate, the body breaks it down into glucose (sugar) and releases the glucose into your bloodstream. With the help of the hormone insulin, the cells of your body then use that glucose as fuel for all the different types of work they have to do.

There are three categories of carbohydrate: starches, sugars, and fiber. Starches and sugars are the main contributors of carbohydrate to our foods. Fiber is also carbohydrate, but its impact on blood glucose can be different than that of other types of carb. There are many types of fiber. (For more information on fiber, see *Fiber and Blood Glucose*, in this chapter.)

You may have heard the terms "simple carbohydrates" and "complex carbohydrates" before. These categories were used for many years to try to explain how various types of carbohydrate affected blood glucose in different ways. These terms are no longer used because recent research suggests that that our old understanding wasn't accurate. We now know that once carbohydrate is broken down, the body doesn't know whether the resulting glucose came from the carbohydrate in mashed potatoes or a piece of apple pie. All carbohydrate becomes glucose—the body's preferred and primary source of energy.

If Carbohydrate Raises Blood Glucose, Should I Follow a Low-Carb Eating Plan?

Once you realize that carbohydrate is the nutrient in foods that raises blood glucose the most, you might jump to the conclusion that people with diabetes should steer clear of foods that contain carbohydrate. But that's incorrect. For starters, any eating plan that drastically restricts a particular food or food group is not realistic in the long term. Restricting carbohydrate would limit foods like fruits, vegetables, and whole grains, which are essential for good nutrition. And your body still needs carbohydrate for energy.

In general, the ADA recommends an eating plan in which about 45–65% of your total daily calories come from carbohydrate. The exact grams of carbohydrate you eat will vary depending on your total calorie goal and a number of other factors.

There's been a lot of talk in recent years about using low-carb meal plans to lose weight. Most of these plans restrict carbohydrate intake to the point where less than 40% of your total daily calories come from carbohydrate. The results from research on these low-carb weight-loss plans have been mixed, and the long-term effectiveness of low-carb eating plans hasn't been shown. At this point, many diabetes experts conclude that there's insufficient evidence to recommend low-carb diets, especially to people with type 2 diabetes. Beyond the question of long-term effectiveness, there are safety concerns about following such a plan over the long term, such as concerns about the progression of heart and kidney problems.

It is most important to consider the total calories that you eat every day if you are considering weight loss, so it can be counterproductive to focus on only whether the calories come from carbohydrate or protein or fat. Therefore, it is best to choose healthy carbohydrate sources, like fruits, vegetables, whole grains, and nonfat and low-fat dairy foods. You do want to limit the not-so-healthy carbohydrate sources, like foods that contain added sugars and sweets, because they contribute concentrated amounts of calories and fats and add little in the way of essential vitamins and minerals.

The best advice? Find a sensible and realistic healthy eating plan for you that is based on sound science. The eating plan should help you lose weight (if you need to) and, even more importantly, keep weight off the rest of your life.

What about Sugars?

First, let's get a few facts straight. Note the plural on "sugars" in the header. The sources of sugars we eat number far more than just the white granular stuff. There are sugars that occur naturally in foods, such as the fructose in fruit and the lactose in milk. Other sugars—such as granulated sugar, brown sugar, and high-fructose corn syrup—are added to foods when they are baked, cooked, prepared, or processed. The most important thing to remember about sugars is that they are carbohydrate and will raise your blood glucose.

IF I HAVE DIABETES, CAN I EAT SUGARY FOODS AND SWEETS?

The short answer is yes. People with diabetes can eat sweets, as long as you account for them in your eating plan and adjust your medications to respond to the extra carbohydrate. Carb counting can help you do this, and you'll learn how in this book. (This may be a surprise—for many years people with diabetes were told to avoid sugar. But now we know that the total amount of carbohydrate in a food or meal is the most important factor.)

This doesn't mean that you should regularly eat candy, cake, and cookies. Realize that even a small serving of these types of foods contain a lot of carbohydrate. Cake and cookies also contain a lot of calories and fat. So you'll want to limit them to special occasions and indulge in small portions, in addition to counting the carbs in your overall carb counting records.

Tips for Eating Fewer Sweets

- Choose a few favorite desserts and decide how often to eat them.
- Satisfy your sweet tooth with a bite or two of your favorite sweet rather than eating the whole thing.
- If you have a difficult time eating smaller portions or how often you eat sweets, it is best not to bring large portions of sweets into your home. You might only order dessert at restaurants or just purchase a small quantity at a time.
- Split a dessert with a dining companion in a restaurant. Ask for several forks or spoons to share the treat.
- Take advantage of smaller portions—kiddie, small, or regular—at ice cream shops or in the supermarket.
- Check your blood glucose from time to time, two to three hours after you eat a sweet to see how high it makes your blood glucose rise.

Easy Ways to Eat Less Sugar

- Instead of regular soda, go for diet soda, seltzer water, or, even better, water.
- When you order or buy iced tea, make sure it is unsweetened or sweetened with a low-calorie sweetener.
- When you buy fruit drinks or flavored seltzers, read the Nutrition Facts label. Make sure the calories, carbohydrate, and sugars are near zero. In general, it's better to drink water and eat fresh fruit.
- Trade canned fruit packed in heavy syrup for fruit packed in its own juice or light syrup.
- Use low-calorie sweeteners instead of sugar.
- Use low- or no-sugar jelly or jam instead of regular.

Fiber and Blood Glucose

As explained earlier, fiber is a type of carbohydrate. There are hundres of different types of fibers in our foods. Depending on which type you eat, fiber can affect blood glucose differently than other carbohydrates. Some fibers can slow down the absorption of glucose, resulting in lower rises in blood glucose after eating. Some fibers are also helpful for weight loss because they make you feel full and satisfied. Fiber has no calories. Fiber is an essential part of a healthy eating plan.

Easy Tips to Fit in Fiber

The U.S. Food and Drug Administration (FDA) defines foods with more than 5 grams of dietary fiber per serving as "excellent" sources, whereas foods that provide between 2.5 and 4.9 grams per serving are considered "good" sources.

Look for these items and check the Nutrition Facts label to see how much fiber a food contains.

• whole-grain cereals, breads, and crackers

• whole grains, such as barley, bulgur, and buckwheat

• beans and peas—these types of foods, called legumes, are great sources of fiber

• fruits and vegetables that are high in fiber, such as acorn and butternut squash, broccoli, carrots, zucchini, berries, plum, prunes, and apples

• nuts and seeds

What Is the Glycemic Index and Should I Use It with Carb Counting?

The glycemic index (GI) is a list of foods that details how various foods affect blood glucose levels. It was developed in the early 1980s by researchers who studied how quickly or slowly various carbohydrate-containing foods raised blood glucose—bread, corn, pasta, beans, fruit, and others. The GI research helped show that not all carbohydrates raise blood glucose levels the same amount.

They showed, for instance, that potatoes raised blood glucose more quickly than fruit and that legumes raised blood glucose quite slowly.

This is valuable information, but it can be difficult for people with diabetes to use the GI for blood glucose control. That's because the GI only evaluates one food at a time. Most people eat several foods in a meal, and some are high in carbohydrate and others are high in protein or fat. The combination of foods in a meal is what determines the effect on blood glucose. In addition, a number of other factors affect how quickly foods raise blood glucose, such as:

- How much blood glucose–lowering medication you take and the type of medication you take
- The fiber content of the foods you eat
- The ripeness of the fruit or vegetable you eat
- Whether the food is cooked or raw
- How quickly or slowly you eat
- The level of blood glucose before a meal (when the starting point is low, blood glucose rises faster after a meal)
- The time of your last dose of diabetes medication and the time you eat

Although the GI may not account for all of this, it can be another tool in your meal planning toolbox. As you progress with carb counting, you may develop your own personal GI. Your records may show that the carbohydrate in certain foods affects your blood glucose more than others. This information can help you fine-tune your blood glucose management.

2

◆ ◆

Basic Carb Counting

There are two levels of carb counting: basic and advanced. Everyone starts at the basic level, so that's where we'll start, too. Later on, you may find that you want or need to progress to the advanced techniques. We'll cover those methods in Chapter 11. For now, let's focus on the basics to get you started.

The focus of basic carb counting is to eat about the same amount of carbohydrate at the same times each day in order to keep your blood glucose levels in your target ranges. The first step is to learn how to count the amount of carbohydrate in different foods.

In This Chapter, You'll Learn:

How to count carbohydrate

How much carbohydrate to eat

If you're ready for carb counting

Two Ways to Count

There are two ways to count carbohydrates: counting grams of carbohydrate and counting carbohydrate servings. Counting carb servings is easier and is usually a close enough estimate for basic carb counting. But there may be times when you need to count grams, so it is best to be aware of both methods.

REMEMBER THE NUMBER 15

If you're counting carb servings, the general rule is that 15 grams of carbohydrate equals one carb serving. The size of the serving will vary depending on the type of food. For example, one carb serving equals

- 1/2 cup of mashed potatoes
- 1 ounce of dry cereal, or
- 1 slice of bread

All of these servings contain 15 grams of carbohydrate. This also means that if you eat more than the serving size of the food, you will need to count more than one serving of carb.

Table 1-1 in Chapter 1 shows examples of common food servings that contain 15 grams of carbohydrate. However, in the real world, not all servings contain exactly 15 grams of carbohydrate. The number will vary from serving to serving, from food to food. There are lots of resources out there to help you figure out grams of carb and serving sizes. As a starting point, refer to Table 2-1 in this chapter. For a more detailed list, see Appendix 1, which lists many commonly eaten foods with the exact number of grams of carbohydrate per serving. As we go on, we'll learn how to find the carbohydrate content on a packaged foods' Nutrition Facts label. There's also a list of books and websites in Appendix 2 that may be helpful.

Table 2-1 Carbohydrate Servings and Grams of Carbohydrate

Carbohydrate Servings	Grams of carbohydrate	Grams of carbohydrate per carbohydrate serving
1/2	6–7	6–7
1	15	8–22
2	30	23–37
3	45	38–52
4	60	53–65
5	75	68–82
6	90	83–95

What are grams of carbohydrate?

Don't confuse gram weight on the serving size of a Nutrition Facts label with carbohydrate grams. Answer these True/False questions to check your knowledge of grams.

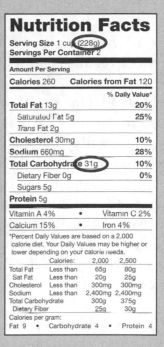

Nutrition Facts

Serving Size 1 cup (228g)
Servings Per Container 2

Amount Per Serving

Calories 260   Calories from Fat 120

	% Daily Value*
Total Fat 13g	**20%**
Saturated Fat 5g	**25%**
Trans Fat 2g	
Cholesterol 30mg	**10%**
Sodium 660mg	**28%**
Total Carbohydrate 31g	**10%**
Dietary Fiber 0g	**0%**
Sugars 5g	
Protein 5g	

Vitamin A 4%	•	Vitamin C 2%
Calcium 15%	•	Iron 4%

*Percent Daily Values are based on a 2,000 calorie diet. Your Daily Values may be higher or lower depending on your calorie needs.

	Calories:	2,000	2,500
Total Fat	Less than	65g	80g
Sat Fat	Less than	20g	25g
Cholesterol	Less than	300mg	300mg
Sodium	Less than	2,400mg	2,400mg
Total Carbohydrate		300g	375g
Dietary Fiber		25g	30g

Calories per gram:
Fat 9   •   Carbohydrate 4   •   Protein 4

1. True   False   A gram is a unit of weight in the metric system.

2. True   False   Carbohydrate is measured in grams (g).

3. True   False   When you weigh something that is 1 ounce (oz), the metric conversion is 30 g.

4. True   False   The weight of a food portion will tell you how many grams of carbohydrate are in it.

Answers: 1. true; 2. true; 3. true; 4. false.
The number of grams of carbohydrate, protein, and fat in a food is not the same as the weight of the food itself. For example, a medium (4 oz) apple may weigh 120 grams (there are 30 grams in an ounce), but the amount of carbohydrate in it is about 15 grams. A medium (6 oz) potato weighs 180 grams (30 grams × 6 oz), but the amount of carbohydrate in it is about 30 grams. However, there are now food scales available that can be programmed to give you a pretty close estimate to the nutrients contained in the food you weigh.

How Much Carbohydrate Should I Eat?

There is no set amount of carbohydrate that is right for everyone. The amount of carbohydrate you need to eat at your meals and snacks should be based on several factors:
- Your height and weight
- Your usual eating habits and daily schedule
- The foods you like to eat

- Your amount of physical activity
- Your health status and diabetes goals
- The diabetes medications you take and the times that you take them
- Your blood glucose monitoring results
- The results of your blood lipid (fat in the bloodstream) tests

To help you determine how much carbohydrate to eat, you need to consider several factors, such as whether you are male or female, small or large, and want to lose weight. As a starting point, most women need three to four carbohydrate servings (45–60 grams) and most men need about four to five carbohydrate servings (60–75 grams) at each meal. You may need less if you want to lose weight. Take a look at Table 2-2 on page 16 to get a general idea of how much carbohydrate you should eat. A dietitian who specializes in diabetes care can help you determine the amount of carbohydrate that best fits your needs (see Chapter 12 for tips on finding a dietitian). When you're using basic carb counting, it is important to keep the amount of carbohydrate you eat at meals and snacks about the same from meal to meal and day to day. This will help you better manage your blood glucose.

Are You Ready to Begin Basic Carb Counting?

We've covered the basics—now it's time for you to decide if you're ready to use basic carb counting as your meal-planning approach. Are you ready to:

1. Find a meal planning approach that fits your lifestyle and desire for more flexibility?   ☐ Yes ☐ No

2. Find a meal planning approach that helps you achieve better control of your blood glucose levels?   ☐ Yes ☐ No

3. Learn more about foods and how much carbohydrate is in them? ☐ Yes ☐ No

4. Pay more attention to what you eat and the amount you eat? ☐ Yes ☐ No

5. Keep food records that detail the types of foods, the amounts of food, when you eat, and how much carb is in each food, meal, or snack? ☐ Yes ☐ No

6. Check blood glucose levels at least two times a day and record the results? For example, select either breakfast, lunch, or dinner; then check before you eat the meal and two hours after the meal. ☐ Yes ☐ No

7. Weigh and measure servings? ☐ Yes ☐ No

8. Read the Nutrition Facts label on packaged foods to find the Total Carbohydrate content? ☐ Yes ☐ No

9. Spend time to learn how much carbohydrate you need to eat to keep your blood glucose levels in control? ☐ Yes ☐ No

10. Use a carb counting book for foods that don't have a label? ☐ Yes ☐ No

Hopefully, you're ready to move forward. There's no doubt that carb counting requires some learning and adjustment—it can be challenging. As time goes on, carb counting will hopefully become easier for you and the process won't seem as rigorous. So let's get started!

Table 2-2 How Much Carbohydrate Should You Eat?

	Women who want to lose weight	Women (older and smaller)	Women (moderate to large size), older men (small to moderate size) who want to lose weight	Children, teen girls, active larger women, men (small to moderate size)	Teen boys, active men (moderate to large size)
Calorie Range[1]	1200–1400 calories	1400–1600 calories	1600–1900 calories	1900–2300 calories	2300–2800 calories
% Calories from carbohydrate[2]	40–45%	40–45%	40–45%	45–50%	45–50%
Carb (g)[3]	130–160	150–180	180–210	215–260	260–300
Carb servings per day (~15 g of carb per carb serving)	8–10	9–11	11–13	13–16	16–19
Servings per day of:					
Grains, beans, and starchy vegetables	4–5	5–6	6–8	8–10	10–12
Fruits	2–3	2–3	3–4	3–4	4–5
Milk[4]	2	2	2	2	2
Vegetables, nonstarchy	3	3	4	4	5
Meats[5]	6 oz	7 oz	8 oz	9 oz	10 oz
Fats	35–40%	35–40%	30–35%	30–35%	30–35%
Fat servings (~5 g of fat in each fat serving)	7	9	10	13	16

[1] The groups of people described in this row are generalizations. To learn how many calories you need, as well as how much of the other nutrients you need to reach your diabetes and nutrition goals, work with a dietitian who specializes in diabetes (see Chapter 12).

[2] For each calorie level, there are two variations for the nutrient breakdown. One calls for 40–45% of calories from carbohydrate and 35–40% of calories from fat. This might be a little high in fat, but some people with type 2 diabetes and lipid problems may find this helpful. Make sure that as much of your fat as possible comes from monounsaturated and polyunsaturated fat sources—think liquid oils versus solid fats. The other variation calls for 45–50% of calories from carbohydrate and 30–35% of calories from fat.

[3] The total grams of carbohydrate and servings of carbohydrate are from grains, beans, starchy vegetables, fruits, and milk. Nonstarchy vegetables aren't counted in the carbohydrate total.

[4] Based on nonfat milk (12 g of carbohydrate and 8 g of protein per 8 oz), according to the 2010 report, *Dietary Reference Intakes for Calcium and Vitamin D*, from the Institute of Medicine of the National Academy of Sciences (www.iom.edu). Children between 9 and 18 years old need 1300 mg of calcium per day. They should get at least 3 servings of milk per day. Adults between 19 and 70 years old need 1000 mg of calcium per day. They should have about 2 servings of milk per day plus another serving of a high source of calcium. Adults older than 70 years of age need 1200 mg of calcium per day. If you don't or can't drink milk, you need to find another source of calcium to meet your nutrition needs. To get an equivalent amount of carbohydrate, add another 24 g from either grains, beans, starchy vegetables, or fruit.

[5] Calculated based on lean meat figures (7 g of protein and 3 g of fat per ounce). Use more or less grams or servings of fat based on the type of meats you tend to eat.

3

◆ ◆

Keeping Track

In a perfect world you would eat about the same amount of carbohydrate at the same times, seven days a week. However, for most people this plan just doesn't mesh with their schedules, and with the medication options available today, people with diabetes have more flexibility in meal planning. Depending on your preferences and your daily routine, you can put together a daily meal plan that works for you.

> **In This Chapter, You'll Learn:**
>
> How to determine your real life eating habits
>
> How to use a food diary and blood glucose records
>
> How to build a personal database of carb counting information

That's why it's important to let your health care providers know as much about your eating style and daily schedule as you can. The best way to accomplish this is to keep records of your current food habits in a food diary. You'll also need to figure out how much carbohydrate you eat and when on most days. Eating similar amounts of carbohydrate on a fairly regular schedule is the cornerstone of basic carb counting. Keep detailed, and honest, records. It's the only way you can trust your results and put them to good use in managing blood glucose.

Your records are particularly important if you take blood glucose–lowering medication, and most people with diabetes do. Your diabetes care providers need to know your preferred schedule of

19

meals and snacks and when you usually eat, because all of these factors affect the type of blood glucose–lowering medication they prescribe for you and the way they teach you to take them. Don't let them prescribe medications for you based on an idealized nine-to-five lifestyle that simply isn't true to your life. Some medications have different have onset and peak times and durations of action. This "action curve" needs to be in sync with when you eat. (For more information on medications and their effects, see Chapter 10.)

Seven Steps

Take a look at these seven steps to help you get a sense of your eating patterns, figure out how much carbohydrate you currently eat and the types of carbohydrate-containing foods you eat, and compare your food records with your blood glucose records. Take these steps one at a time and you'll be well on your way with carb counting.

STEP 1: KEEP FOOD RECORDS

Begin keeping a food diary by recording the foods you eat at breakfast, lunch, and dinner. Don't forget to include snacks and nibbles. Yes, crumbs do count! Keep these records for a full week, including the weekend. It's important to note both the type of food and the amount that you eat. The more accurate you can be, the more helpful your food records will be to you and to your health care provider. It helps to use a food scale and measuring cups and spoons to measure portions accurately, especially as you're learning. You can design your own food record or use one similar to the record on Table 3-1. Your food records should include the following:
- Day of the week
- Mealtime
- Amounts of food
- Carb grams for each food
- Total carb grams for the meal or snack

Begin by just entering the food you ate for two days.

Table 3-1 Sample Food Diary

Day	Meal	Food	Amount	Carbs
Monday				
	Breakfast (7am)	Blueberry bagel	1 medium (3.7 oz)	
		Light cream cheese	2 Tbsp	
		Strawberries	1 cup, sliced	
	TOTAL			
	Lunch (noon)	Thin-crust cheese pizza (14″)	3 slices	
		Garden salad	1 1/2 cups	
		Thousand Island dressing	2 Tbsp	
		Frozen yogurt, low-fat	1/2 cup	
		Sugar cone	1	
	TOTAL			
	Dinner (6:30pm)	Grilled chicken breast strips	5 oz, cooked	
		Barbecue sauce	2 Tbsp	
		Long-grain brown rice	1 cup	
		Corn on the cob	1 large	
		Margarine	2 Tbsp	
		Applesauce (no sugar added)	1 cup	
	TOTAL			
	Snack (9pm)	Oatmeal raisin cookie	1 large (2.5 oz)	
	TOTAL			

Table 3-1 Sample Food Diary (continued)

Day	Meal	Food	Amount	Carbs
Tuesday				
	Breakfast (9am)	Raisin bran muffin	1 (4.5 oz)	
		Orange juice	8 oz	
		Milk, nonfat	8 oz	
	TOTAL			
	Lunch (12:30pm)	Chicken pot pie	8 oz	
		Dinner roll	1	
		Apple, medium	6 oz	
	TOTAL			
	Dinner (7:45pm)	Spaghetti	2 cups	
		Meat sauce	3/4 cup	
		Parmesan cheese	2 Tbsp	
		Garden salad	1 cup	
		French dressing, fat-free	2 Tbsp	
	TOTAL			
	Snack (10:30pm)	Ice cream, light	1 cup	
		Blueberries	1/2 cup	
	TOTAL			

STEP 2: FIND THE FOODS YOU ATE THAT CONTAIN CARBOHYDRATE

After you have one week of your food diary completed, go through and circle the foods that contain carbohydrate. You can identify these foods by using the list of foods in Appendix 1 or by using one or more of the resources listed in Appendix 2. See Table 3-2 for an example. As you can see, it's not just the rice, bread, and desserts; dairy foods and fruits contain carb, and even salad dressing may contain a few grams.

Table 3-2 Sample Food Diary

Day	Meal	Food	Amount	Carbs
Monday				
	Breakfast (7am)	Blueberry bagel	1 medium (3.7 oz)	
		Light cream cheese	2 Tbsp	
		Strawberries	1 cup, sliced	
	TOTAL			
	Lunch (noon)	Thin-crust cheese pizza (14")	3 slices	
		Garden salad	1 1/2 cups	
		Thousand Island dressing	2 Tbsp	
		Frozen yogurt, low-fat	1/2 cup	
		Sugar cone	1	
	TOTAL			
	Dinner (6:30pm)	Grilled chicken breast strips	5 oz, cooked	
		Barbecue sauce	2 Tbsp	
		Long-grain brown rice	1 cup	
		Corn on the cob	1 large	
		Margarine	2 Tbsp	
		Applesauce (no sugar added)	1 cup	
	TOTAL			
	Snack (9pm)	Oatmeal raisin cookie	1 large (2.5 oz)	
	TOTAL			

Table 3-2 Sample Food Diary (continued)

Day	Meal	Food	Amount	Carbs
Tuesday				
	Breakfast (9am)	Raisin bran muffin	1 (4.5 oz)	
		Orange juice	8 oz	
		Milk, nonfat	8 oz	
	TOTAL			
	Lunch (12:30pm)	Chicken pot pie	8 oz	
		Dinner roll	1	
		Apple, medium	6 oz	
	TOTAL			
	Dinner (7:45pm)	Spaghetti	2 cups	
		Meat sauce	3/4 cup	
		Parmesan cheese	2 Tbsp	
		Garden salad	1 cup	
		French dressing, fat-free	2 Tbsp	
	TOTAL			
	Snack (10:30pm)	Ice cream, light	1 cup	
		Blueberries	1/2 cup	
	TOTAL			

STEP 3: FIGURE HOW MUCH CARB YOU EAT

Now, go back and figure out the number of grams of carbohydrate in each of the foods you ate. Table 3-3 shows an example of how this is done. Then add up the totals for each meal and snack. If you plan to use carb servings rather than grams of carbohydrate, remember that each carb serving contains about 15 grams (g) of carbohydrate.

Table 3-3 Sample Food Diary

Day	Meal	Food	Amount	Carbs
Monday				
	Breakfast (7am)	Blueberry bagel	1 medium (3.7 oz)	58
		Light cream cheese	2 Tbsp	2
		Strawberries	1 cup, sliced	13
	TOTAL			*73*
	Lunch (noon)	Thin-crust cheese pizza (14")	3 slices	50
		Garden salad	1 1/2 cups	7
		Thousand Island dressing	2 Tbsp	5
		Frozen yogurt, low-fat	1/2 cup	23
		Sugar cone	1	8
	TOTAL			*93*
	Dinner (6:30pm)	Grilled chicken breast strips	5 oz, cooked	0
		Barbecue sauce	2 Tbsp	4
		Long-grain brown rice	1 cup	45
		Corn on the cob	1 large	32
		Margarine	2 Tbsp	0
		Applesauce (no sugar added)	1 cup	28
	TOTAL			*109*
	Snack (9pm)	Oatmeal raisin cookie	1 large (2.5 oz)	32
	TOTAL			*32*

Table 3-3 Sample Food Diary (continued)

Day	Meal	Food	Amount	Carbs
Tuesday				
	Breakfast (9am)	Raisin bran muffin	1 (4.5 oz)	60
		Orange juice	8 oz	25
		Milk, nonfat	8 oz	12
	TOTAL			97
	Lunch (12:30pm)	Chicken pot pie	8 oz	45
		Dinner roll	1	14
		Apple, medium	6 oz	25
	TOTAL			84
	Dinner (7:45pm)	Spaghetti	2 cups	90
		Meat sauce	3/4 cup	15
		Parmesan cheese	2 Tbsp	0
		Garden salad	1 cup	6
		French dressing, fat-free	2 Tbsp	12
	TOTAL			123
	Snack (10:30pm)	Ice cream, light	1 cup	40
		Blueberries	1/2 cup	11
	TOTAL			51

STEP 4: SIT BACK AND OBSERVE

Now use the information in your food diary to see if you eat about the same amount of carbohydrate for breakfast, lunch, dinner, and snacks each day, and if you eat at the same times each day. In the two days of sample records on pages 25–26, the carbohydrate in the breakfasts vary from 73 to 97 grams, and the breakfast times are very different, too. One day breakfast is at 7 a.m. and the next it's at 9 a.m. As you have already learned, varying the amount of carbohydrate and the timing of breakfast this much will make it more difficult to control blood glucose levels. That's particularly true if you, like most people, take the same amount of medication each day.

STEP 5: GET FAMILIAR WITH THE CARB COUNTS OF THE FOODS YOU EAT

Most of us are creatures of habit—we eat the same foods day in and day out. That's good news when it comes to carb counting because this makes it easier to build your own personal "database" of carb counts.

As you start to build your personal database, think about what record-keeping format works for you (a sample is found in Appendix 3). Will it be best to keep your database in your smartphone, or in a small notebook that you carry with you? Or is it better for you to keep it as a continually growing spreadsheet on your computer, with the type of information in Table 3-4: the food, the amount you eat in a serving, and the carb count in grams? You be the judge.

Table 3-4 Sample Personal Database— My Common Meals and Snacks

Meal	Serving (amount I eat)	Grams of carbohydrate*
Breakfast 1: (at home)		
Honey Nut Cheerios	1 cup	24
All Bran with Extra Fiber	1/2 cup	23
Milk, nonfat	1 cup	12
Blueberries	1/2 cup	10
Total		69
Breakfast 2: (in the car)		
Whole-wheat toast (for egg sandwich)	2 slices	26
Egg (fried)	1 large	0
Cheddar cheese, reduced-fat	1 oz	0
Banana	1 medium (4 oz)	27
Total		53
Lunch 1:		
Whole-wheat bread	2 slices	26
Smoked turkey, sliced	2 oz	0
Swiss cheese, part-skim	1 oz	1
Baby carrots	7–10	8
Grape tomatoes	5–8	3
Apple, Granny Smith	1 large (7 oz)	29
Total		66

*Nutrition Information obtained from www.ars.usda.gov/nutrientdata (the USDA searchable database. For more information about this database see Appendix 2) and Nutrition Facts labels.

Start to build your carbohydrate database by making a list of the foods you regularly eat at meals. Then determine the carb counts for one serving of each food on the list. When you have a Nutrition Facts label, use the Total Carbohydrate count from the package. If the size of the serving you eat is bigger or smaller, do the math to determine the carb count for the amount you eat. When you don't have a Nutrition Facts label to work from, such as with fresh fruits and vegetables, look up carb counts in Appendix 1 or in one of many available resources listed in Appendix 2.

Carb counts: From foods to meals

After you have looked up the carb counts of the individual foods you regularly eat, count up the total grams of carbohydrate in meals that you regularly eat. Keep a record of these as well. Again, we are creatures of habit, not only in the foods we choose to eat, but in the way we combine these foods for meals and the amount of food we eat. You can save time in the long run by spending a few minutes developing a database of the carb counts of your common meals.

STEP 6: FIGURE OUT HOW MUCH CARB YOU SHOULD EAT

Now you have a picture of how much carbohydrate you usually eat at your meals and snacks. Now you need to determine whether the amount you're eating is too much, too little, or just about right. As we said before, your target carbohydrate intake will vary based on a variety of factors. Most women need three to four carbohydrate servings (45–60 g) and most men need about four to five carbohydrate servings (60–75 g) at each meal.

STEP 7: MATCH UP WHAT YOU EAT WITH BLOOD GLUCOSE RECORDS

The next step is to match your food records with your blood glucose records. Checking your blood glucose at various times of the day is the best way to learn how your blood glucose responds to food, activity, stress, and other things in your life. But it's equally important to record the results! If you don't record the results, the data—and the opportunity to learn from it—are lost.

After-meal blood glucose checks are especially important, particularly as you are learning carb counting. That's because after-meal (one and a half to two hours after the time you begin eating) blood glucose checks help you see the impact of the carbohydrate you ate on your blood glucose. Obviously, your goal is to have your blood glucose in target ranges both before meals and after as often as possible. Table 1-2 (page 5) gives you the target ranges of blood glucose, so you can see where yours are in relation to them.

Now don't be alarmed; you don't need to check your blood glucose constantly! To observe the ups and downs in your blood glucose, yet avoid feeling like a human pincushion, set up a rotating blood glucose checking pattern. Check your blood glucose two to three times a day at different times on different days. In just a few days, you'll have results from around the clock. Table 3-5 shows a four-day sample pattern with two checks a day.

Table 3-5 Sample Schedule for Blood Glucose Checks

	Fasting	1–2 hrs after break-fast	Before lunch	1–2 hrs after lunch	Before dinner	1–2 hrs after dinner	Bed	Other
Day 1	X	X						
Day 2			X	X				
Day 3					X	X		
Day 4	X							X

You'll likely need to check your blood glucose levels more often when you start carb counting, until you get a sense of your blood glucose patterns. You might also have to check more if you make a change in the dose of a medication, add a medication, start an exercise program, etc. When your diabetes management plan changes, more frequent blood glucose checks can help you adjust.

Keeping Records for the Long Haul

Following this seven-step plan for a few days helps you get a sense of how carb counting works and how your blood glucose level reacts to the food you eat. Going forward, you'll want to keep even more detailed records to help you and your diabetes care provider track your progress and make adjustments to your treatment plan. For your long-term record keeping, you'll want to note more than just your carbohydrate intake and blood glucose levels. The information below introduces other factors you'll want to track:

PHYSICAL ACTIVITY

Being physically active generally lowers blood glucose (but be aware that it can also raise blood glucose). Being physically active is an important part of managing your diabetes, and an important part of staying healthy. If you're not already physically active, it's always a good idea to start! Any amount of activity is good—but it's also important to remember to note it in your records. Be sure to write down the type of activity, how long you did it, and when. Be sure to check with your health care team before you start an exercise regimen.

EMOTIONS, STRESS, ILLNESS, AND UNUSUAL SITUATIONS

Changes in day-to-day events can affect blood glucose levels, too. When you or a loved one is ill or when you're dealing with a deadline at work or with conflict in a relationship, you may see changes in your results. It's important to record information about the emotions you're feeling and the stressful situations you're dealing with. It's also important to record positive emotions and situations. For example, vacations may be a positive change to your regular routine, but vacations also often cause you to eat differently and at different times. Women should note menstrual periods in their records as well; the various phases of the menstrual cycle, including the hormonal surges of adolescence and menopause, can affect blood glucose levels.

MEDICATIONS

If you take blood glucose–lowering medications, it's important for you to track the medications you take, how much, and when. This information, along with all the other factors in your records, will help fine-tune your diabetes control.

Keep It All in One Place

Most people find it easier to keep one record that includes space for all of the factors that affect blood glucose, all in one place. Unfortunately, most of the blood glucose records that come with glucose meters or other diabetes supplies don't provide enough room. We encourage you to try using the record form in Appendix 3 or the sample form in Table 3-6 on page 32–33. Of course, you can use this sample as a starting point and make any changes you want to fit your needs. A recording form should provide room for:

- The timing of your meals and snacks
- The types and doses of your diabetes medications
- The foods you eat, including the amount and the grams of carbohydrate or number of carb servings
- The results of your blood glucose checks, with a note of the time of the check
- An "other" column to record the type and amount of your physical activity
- Your daily schedule
- Illnesses, emotions, or stressful situations
- Other reasons why your blood glucose results might have been different from what you expected
- You can also record information about activity, emotions, and general observations under a "notes" section.

Table 3-6 Carb Counting and Blood Glucose Record

Day/Date: Tuesday, June 3 (I:Carb Ratio = 1 unit to 12 g of carb)

| Time/meal | Diabetes medicines | | Food | | Carb grams |
	Type	Amount	Type	Amount	
6:45 a	Lispro	8 units			
7 a/ breakfast			Shredded Wheat 'n Bran with	1/2 cup	20
			Cheerios	3/4 cup	17
			Milk	1 cup	12
			Banana	1 medium	20
					Total 69
12:30 p	Lispro	7 units	Sub sandwich— 6" turkey, ham, cheese, lettuce, tomato, onions, pickles, mustard	1	46
			Pretzels	2.5 oz bag	34
					Total 80
5:00 p/ Snack	Lispro	2 units	Apple	8 oz/1 lg	30
7:15 p	Lispro	9 units			
dinner			Macaroni and cheese, prepared with sliced turkey sausage	1.5 cups	98
			Broccoli, steamed	1 cup	8
			Fruit cup	3/4 cup	22
10:30 p bedtime	Glargine 22 units				

Notes about day:
Went for a walk after dinner
Blood glucose has gotten low right before bed several times recently.

Blood glucose results							
Fasting/ before b'fast/ time	After b'fast/ time	Before lunch/ time	After lunch/ time	Before dinner/ time	After dinner/ time	Before bed/ time	Other/ time
92/ 6:30 a	210/ 8:45 a						
		89/ 12:30 p	154/ 2:00 p				
		126/ 7:00 p	205/ 9:00 p				Checked at 11 p, felt low, BG=65

Meet Jane

Jane is a 45-year-old schoolteacher who was recently diagnosed with type 2 diabetes. She takes 500 mg of metformin before breakfast and dinner. She feels she gets enough physical activity at work. She is interested in basic carb counting as a way to help her keep her blood glucose in control but also so she can have flexibility with the food choices she makes.

She checks her blood glucose when she gets up and does a second check at various times before and after meals. One day she checks after lunch and the next day after dinner, but always within one to two hours after she starts to eat. Her blood glucose readings after lunch are 140–175 mg/dl, within her target range after meals. But the ones after dinner are in the 200–230 mg/dl range, and she is concerned about this. By looking at the information in her record, she realizes that she's eating about 60 grams of carb at lunch and 110 grams at dinner and that she is not active in the evenings. After lunch, she is teaching and on her feet and moving for three more hours. But when she gets home, she fixes dinner and then watches her favorite TV shows.

Keeping records helped Jane see how the amount of carbohydrate she eats and her activity level has an effect on her blood glucose. She realizes she needs to balance the amount of carbohydrate she eats each day by eating more at lunch when she is active and less in the evening. She and her dietitian set a goal of 45–60 grams of carbohydrate at both lunch and dinner.

You can see Jane's record in Table 3-7 on pages 36–37.

Table 3-7 Jane's Carb Counting and Blood Glucose Record

Day/Date: Tuesday, January 23

Time/meal	Diabetes medicines Type	Amount	Food Type	Amount	Carb grams
6:00 a	met-formin	500 mg			
6:15 a/ breakfast			Frozen waffles	2	29
			Maple syrup	2 Tbsp	26
			Raspberries	1/2	8
			Yogurt with fruit, nonfat with low-cal sweetener	1 medium	20
					Total 83
12:30 p/ lunch			Chunky split-pea and ham soup	1 11-oz can	33
			Ritz crackers	5	9
			Pear	1 6 oz	22
					Total 64
6:00 p/ dinner	met-formin	500 mg	Pork chop, baked	3 oz	0
			Mashed potatoes with butter	1 cup	33
			Green peas	1/2 cup	15
			Dinner roll with butter	1 tsp	15 0
			Apple pie	1/8 9" pie	43
					Total 106

Notes about day:
On my feet and moving while teaching after lunch for 3 hours.

Blood glucose results							
Fasting/before b'fast/time	After b'fast/time	Before lunch/time	After lunch/time	Before dinner/time	After dinner/time	Before bed/time	Other/time
90/ 6:00 a							
			165/ 2:00 p				
				116/ 6:00 p	223/ 8:00 p		

4

◆ ◆

Protein, Fat, and Alcohol Count, Too

Carb counting focuses on the foods you eat that contain carbohydrate. It's true that the protein and fat in foods, when you eat them in recommended amounts, have little effect on blood glucose levels. However, you cannot ignore foods that contain protein and fat. Here are the reasons why:

1. Protein and fat contain calories, and all calories count. Protein and fat might not affect your blood glucose levels much, but if you eat too much of them, they can add to your waistline.
2. Too much protein, especially animal protein, and too much fat, especially saturated fat and trans fat, are not healthy for anyone—but especially for people with diabetes.
3. The fat and protein in your meals may slow down the rise in blood glucose. When you eat a meal that is higher in protein than usual—for example, an 8-ounce steak or prime rib—your blood glucose might rise more slowly than you expect. In addition, when you eat a meal that is higher in fat than usual—for example, fried chicken, mashed potatoes, and gravy followed by a piece of cheesecake for dessert—your blood glucose might rise more slowly and peak later than you expect. You need to

know about these differences and account for them while you manage your blood glucose levels.

The Need for Protein and Fat

Our bodies need some protein to build muscles. Protein is made up of amino acids that the body needs in order to work properly. Our bodies also need some fat, to carry the fat-soluble vitamins A, D, E, and K; cushion the body's vital organs; and provide insulation to keep us warm. But most people consume more protein and fat than the body needs to conduct its business, and many people choose to eat less-healthy protein and fat sources.

Which Foods Contain Protein?

Many people would answer "red meat, poultry, and seafood," which is correct. But actually, protein turns up in other foods, too. Many of these other sources contain a combination of protein and carbohydrate or protein and fat. For example, dried beans and peas contain protein and carbohydrate. Nuts contain protein and fat. There are also a variety of soy-based proteins on the market, which are usually lower in fat than meat, but also contain carbohydrate.

Which Foods Contain Fat?

Some foods are just about 100% fat, such as butter, margarine, oil, or regular salad dressing. These foods are often added to other foods to make them taste better—that's why we call them "added fats." On average, one serving of these types of foods contains about 5 grams of fat and 45 calories. Other foods, such as meats, cheese, nuts, whole-milk dairy foods, and most desserts, get some (but not all) of their calories from fat. You might call these "attached fats," where fat is naturally part of the food. In fat-containing foods, the fat is made up of varying amounts of three types of fat—saturated, polyunsaturated, and monounsaturated. (There is also a fourth type, trans fatty acids, or trans fats, found mostly in processed foods, which are also a type of saturated fat. We'll talk more about trans fats in a bit.) Here is some information on the different fats, how they act in the body, and examples of food sources of each.

Monounsaturated Fats

Actions: lower total cholesterol and LDL and HDL cholesterols

Sources: Oils (liquid canola, olive, peanut)

Polyunsaturated Fats

There are two types of polyunsaturated fats—omega-3s and omega-6s.

Actions of omega-3: Lower risk for heart disease by decreasing stickiness of blood platelets and lowering triglyceride levels.

Sources: Fatty fish, such as salmon, sardines, herring, and albacore tuna
Flax (ground) and flaxseed oil, soybean oil, and canola oil
Walnuts

Actions of omega-6: Lower total cholesterol and LDL cholesterol. They also lower HDL (good) cholesterol, which isn't a benefit.

Sources: Oils (liquid corn, safflower, soybean)

Saturated Fats

Action: Raise total and LDL cholesterol

Sources: Beef, pork, poultry
Butter
Cream cheese
Whole-milk dairy foods

TRANS FATS DEFINED

A small amount of trans fats are found naturally in foods, such as meats and dairy foods. But most trans fats are created through a manufacturing process called partial hydrogenation. Partial hydrogenation takes an unsaturated fat and makes it more saturated—or solid. Think of a margarine made from liquid corn oil and formed into a stick. Food manufacturers use partial hydrogenation to create the more solid form of fat that increases the shelf life of products. Research shows that even small amounts of trans fats raise LDL or "bad" cholesterol and lower HDL or "good" cholesterol.

Health authorities have worked hard to raise awareness of trans fats in recent years, and many food manufacturers have responded by removing or reducing the amount of trans fats in their foods. Still, it's a good idea to be on the lookout for trans fats and to take steps to limit your intake as much as possible. Here are some steps you can take to reduce the amount of trans fats in your eating plan:

- Limit your intake of foods with partially hydrogenated fat, such as margarine, cookies, crackers, fried snack foods, frozen convenience foods, and fried restaurant foods.
- Take advantage of new foods that do not contain trans fats, such as newer margarines and salad dressings.
- Lower your intake of total fat and saturated fat. This will automatically reduce your intake of trans fat.

Watch the Nutrition Facts label, too. Food manufacturers are required to provide data about trans fats under the fat information heading on the label. However, foods that contain less than 0.5 grams of trans fats per serving can be labeled "trans fats free." Double check the ingredients list for things like hydrogenated or partially hydrogenated oils to ensure that you're keeping your trans fat intake as low as possible.

What Does Protein Do to Blood Glucose?

A high-protein meal—which often is high in both protein and fat—may delay the rise of blood glucose in people with type 2 diabetes. If you are used to eating 3–4 ounces of meat at dinner and then on a rare occasion you eat an 8-ounce sirloin, you might find that when you check your blood glucose level one to two hours later, it's not as high as you thought it would be. Then if you check it three to four hours later, when you thought it would be headed down, it may be higher than you expected.

For many years it was thought that about 50% of the protein we ate was "converted" into glucose and that protein just raised blood glucose more slowly than carbohydrate. This theory encouraged health care providers to teach people with diabetes to always eat protein in combination with carbohydrate. Newer research proves that this is not correct. Some people, however, feel they have better blood glucose control and feel more satisfied between meals when they have some protein at each meal. Other people feel that protein in a bedtime snack is helpful, and still others don't think the added protein makes a difference. Find out what works best for you.

The best advice for learning how your body reacts is to monitor your blood glucose several times in the hours after you eat meals or foods that are higher in protein and fat. For instance, you might want to check your blood glucose both two hours and three hours after the meal rather than just two hours after. At two hours, you might not have seen the full impact of the high protein and fat on your blood glucose level. Learn how your body responds to these meals so you can determine a plan to manage them.

For People with Type 1 Diabetes

In people with type 1 diabetes, protein has little effect on blood glucose, unless it is eaten in very large portions; large portions of protein can increase blood glucose and cause a need for more insulin. For people who take oral diabetes medications, adjusting one dose of the medication won't help reduce the rise in blood glucose.

How Much Protein Should You Eat?

The ADA recommends getting 15–20% of your daily calories from protein. The Recommended Daily Allowance (RDA) for the average male is about 60–65 grams of protein and for the average female about 50–55 grams of protein. If you translate this into servings of protein, that's two to three 3-ounce servings of cooked meat or meat substitutes per day. Each ounce of protein food contains about 7 grams of protein. So, a 3-ounce cooked serving has 21 grams. That is a piece of meat about the size of the palm of your hand or a deck of playing cards. The amount of fat and calories in that protein serving will vary, depending on the type of protein you choose (see Table 4-1).

Table 4-1 Fat and Calories for Meat Servings

Type of meat (3 ounces, cooked)	Fat (grams)	Calories
Lean meat (tenderloin, chicken, flounder)	9	165
Medium-fat meats (ground beef, pork chops)	15	225
High-fat meats (country pork ribs)	24	300

What Is Important about Fat and Diabetes?

One of the most important nutrition recommendations for people with diabetes is to eat less saturated fat. That's because saturated fat contributes to heart disease, and people with diabetes already have a two to four times greater risk of developing heart disease than people without diabetes.

Many people with diabetes, especially type 2 diabetes, have abnormal blood fat, or lipid, levels. Blood lipids include cholesterol (total, HDL, and LDL) and triglycerides. The most common blood lipid profile in people with type 2 diabetes is low HDL (sometimes referred to as "good") cholesterol and high triglyceride levels—a combination that increases cardiovascular risks significantly. The ADA recommends that adults with diabetes have their blood fats checked every year. Refer to Table 4-2 for blood fat goals for people with diabetes.

The best way to reduce this risk is to reduce your intake of saturated fat, trans fat, total fat, and cholesterol. Here are some tips:
- Choose reduced-fat, low-fat, or nonfat milk, cheeses, yogurt, and other dairy foods.
- Prepare foods in low-fat ways, such as by sautéing or broiling.
- Eat small portions.
- Choose leaner cuts of red meat, such as flank steak, and white meat poultry without the skin.

Table 4-2 Blood Fat Goals

LDL ("bad") cholesterol	<100 mg/dl
HDL ("good") cholesterol	>40 mg/dl for men, >50 mg/dl for women
Triglycerides (another type of blood fat)	<150 mg/dl

From the ADA's *Standards of Medical Care for Diabetes—2011*.

General nutrition recommendations call for getting between 20% and 35% of calories from total fat. The majority of your fat calories should come from healthier sources, like monounsaturated and polyunsaturated fats. Saturated fat should still not account for more than 7% of your total calories, and trans fats should be kept as near to zero as possible. Also, try to eat no more than 200 mg of cholesterol per day. These guidelines can be a tall order. Approach making changes in your eating habits step by step.

WHAT CAN YOU LEARN FROM THE GRAMS OF TOTAL FAT?

Do you want to know how to figure how much total fat and the types of fats you need? Knowing this information will be helpful when you shop, read labels, and plan meals. Here's an example using a meal plan that calls for 1,500 daily calories with 30% of those calories coming from fat.

Total number of calories:	1,500
Multiply calories by 30%:	1,500
	× .30
	450 calories from fat

Because there are 9 calories in each gram of fat, divide the calories from fat by 9:

$$450 \div 9 = 50 \text{ grams of total fat}$$

Therefore, this meal plan suggests you eat less than 50 grams of fat per day. Recommendations also state that less than 7% of your total calories should come from saturated fat. Now you can also figure out that number, too.

Multiply calories by 07%:	1,500
	× .07
	105 calories from fat

Divide this number by 9 (9 calories per gram of fat):

$$105 \div 9 = 12 \text{ grams of saturated fat}$$

A NOTE ABOUT REDUCED-FAT AND FAT-FREE PRODUCTS

The push to eat less fat has led to the availability of reduced-fat, low-fat, and fat-free versions of foods, such as ice cream, sour cream, cream cheese, salad dressing, potato chips, and margarine. When fat is removed from food to lower the fat content and calories, food manufacturers put "fat replacers" into the products to make them taste good. Fat replacers may be made from carbohydrate, protein, or fat, but the majority of fat replacers in use today are made of carbohydrate. So the calories and fat in the food may be lower—but the carbohydrate content usually is higher. For people with diabetes, these extra grams of carbohydrate can affect blood glucose levels.

If you want to try some of these products, read the Total Carbohydrate listing on the Nutrition Facts labels to determine their carbohydrate content. Try a few. Find ones that you enjoy and help you achieve your nutrition goals. If you don't like them, don't use them—there are plenty of other, good-tasting ways to lower your fat intake.

What about Alcohol?

Alcohol is not food, but it does contain calories, and some alcoholic beverages, such as regular beer, contain carbohydrate. The calories in most alcoholic drinks come from the alcohol, and calories from alcohol are actually more concentrated than the calories from carbohydrate. Alcohol has 7 calories per gram versus 4 calories per gram of carbohydrate. So, the calories from alcohol can add up quickly.

The most important general message about alcohol is to "drink in moderation." General health guidelines and the ADA recommend no more than one drink a day for women and two drinks a day for men. The definition of "one drink" can vary by type, but generally it amounts to 12 ounces of beer, 5 ounces of wine, or 1 1/2 ounces of distilled spirits (liquor).

Alcohol is unique because it can do opposite things in people with diabetes—it can both lower and raise blood glucose levels. It can lower blood glucose levels because it can decrease the amount of glucose released by the liver, and the calories in alcohol do not convert to glucose. You can see how these effects of alcohol, combined with a dose of insulin or other blood glucose–lowering medicine that can cause hypoglycemia, can produce a double whammy effect on your blood glucose levels. When you drink alcohol and take a blood glucose–lowering medication that can cause hypoglycemia, it is critical to eat a sufficient amount of food to avoid dangerously low blood glucose levels. People can have problems with low blood glucose from alcohol a number of hours after drinking and/or overnight.

However, alcoholic drinks that contain carbohydrate, such as regular beer and wine, can increase blood glucose levels. This is caused by the carbohydrate in the beverage, not the alcohol. Do some research—most beers show their carbohydrate content on the label, and there is a move afoot to require all alcoholic drinks to provide nutrition facts. Appendix 1 also lists various types of alcohol with serving sizes and grams of carbohydrate.

How to Drink Alcohol Safely

1. Know your blood glucose. Don't drink if your blood glucose is too low. If you have been drinking, do not drive.

2. Eat a carbohydrate-containing food that will raise your blood glucose and prevent low blood glucose before, during, and/or after you drink.

3. If you drink in the evening, check your blood glucose before you go to bed. If it seems to be decreasing, eat or drink something that contains carbohydrate.

4. If you drink alcohol that does contain carbohydrate, such as regular beer; mixed drinks with fruit juice, soda, or other carbohydrate-containing ingredients; or a liqueur, count these grams of carbohydrate as part of your daily carbohydrate allotment.

5. Be aware that exercise and alcohol within hours of each other can intensify each element's impact on blood glucose. If you exercise and drink alcohol in the same day, monitor your blood glucose carefully.

6. Checking your blood glucose and keeping track of how much and what you drink will help you learn your body's reaction to alcohol.

7. The most important message is to drink in moderation and responsibly.

5

◆ ◆

Weighing and Measuring Foods: A Key to Your Success

Even if you eat only "healthy foods," you can still have blood glucose control problems—and you can still gain weight or struggle to lose weight. It is possible to eat too much healthy food, like whole-grain breads and cereals, fruits, and vegetables. The bottom line is, it's not just a matter of what you eat, it's also a matter of how much.

The extra carbohydrate from servings that are just a bit too large can add up quickly. If, for example, you regularly eat

> **In This Chapter, You'll Learn:**
>
> How to practice portion control
>
> How to weigh and measure food servings
>
> Tips for estimating serving sizes

an extra half cup of pasta or potatoes at dinner, then you're taking in an extra 15 grams of carbohydrate at the meal. If you have a large apple rather than a medium apple at lunch, that's about 10 grams of extra carbohydrate you're eating.

But it's not just the carbohydrate: it might be an extra ounce or two of meat (protein and fat) at dinner and an extra tablespoon of regular salad dressing (fat) at lunch. It is easy to tell yourself that these extras are too small to keep you from achieving blood glucose control, weight loss, or your other diabetes goals. After all, you're not eating a candy bar or a slice of cheesecake! That is true, but extra servings on a daily basis can mean the difference between hitting your blood glucose targets—and/or losing weight—and not.

49

Our Super-Sized Society

In today's society, it is a challenge to manage portion sizes because we are surrounded by ever-larger dinner plates, super-sized fast food meals, and all-you-can-eat buffet restaurants. As time has passed, we've lost sight of reasonable portions. Restaurants commonly serve 10-ounce steaks, two cups of pasta, and three-egg omelets. Clearly, these portions don't follow the serving sizes that we see on food Nutrition Facts labels or the servings suggested in this book. To get your portion sizes under control, you'll sometimes need to weigh and measure your foods to visualize what healthy serving sizes really look like.

How to Measure Servings

If you cook and bake regularly, you're already familiar with common measurements and measurement tools. If you don't, Table 5-1 can help you get comfortable with common weights and measures.

Table 5-1 Common Household Measurements

3 teaspoons (tsp)	=	1 tablespoon (Tbsp)		
4 Tbsp	=	1/4 cup	=	2 fluid ounces
8 Tbsp	=	1/2 cup	=	4 fluid ounces
16 Tbsp	=	1 cup	=	8 fluid ounces
1 cup	=	1/2 pint	=	8 fluid ounces
2 cups	=	1 pint	=	16 fluid ounces
1 ounce	=	30 grams (dry)		

Most people already have the tools they need to measure their servings at home. But there are a few things that you might not have that can be very helpful. You should use these tools as often as possible, until you can look at a serving size and correctly estimate its size.

MEASURING SPOONS

Don't use your regular silverware for measuring foods. They vary in size based on style and won't give you exact measurements. Use a set of measuring spoons for cooking, which usually includes a 1/2 teaspoon, 1 teaspoon, 1/2 tablespoon, and 1 tablespoon. Tip: 3 tsp = 1 Tbsp.

MEASURING CUPS—LIQUIDS

Use a clear glass or plastic 1- or 2-cup measuring cup so you can see through it. It should have lines showing 1/4-, 1/3-, 1/2-, 2/3-, and 3/4-cup measurements. To measure liquids correctly, set the cup down on a flat surface, and look at the markings at eye level to make sure the liquid reaches the proper line.

MEASURING CUPS—SOLIDS

You should have a set that includes 1/4-, 1/2-, 3/4-, and 1-cup measuring cups. Choose the correct size for your serving and fill it to the top. Level the contents of the measuring cup with the flat edge of a knife. For instance, if you need 1/2 cup of uncooked hot cereal, measure it in a 1/2-cup measure and level it off with a flat knife to remove excess.

FOOD SCALE

Food scales vary widely in price and functionality, but you can get a simple one for under $10. You will mainly use it to measure foods that you measure in ounces, such as fresh fruit, bagels, potatoes, snack foods, cereals, baked goods, meats, fish, and cheese. More expensive scales are available, but they are not necessary. On the low end, a food scale will just measure ounces, pounds, grams, and kilograms. On the high end are digital scales that give you an exact measurement with a numeric digital readout rather than making you read between the lines on an analog dial. There are also scales that actually give you the gram weight of the food and the grams of carbohydrate in that amount of the food.

SPECIALIZED ITEMS

If you are just getting started with portion control or are having a difficult time controlling your portions, there are specialized tools available for you. There are plates that are divided into separate sections to help ensure that you're eating proper portion sizes. You can buy bowls that have measurement markings on them, so you know exactly how much of a food you are eating when you fill the bowl. There are even food dispensers that release a set amount of food with a twist of a dial. New products are being released all the time to make measuring healthy serving sizes easy and achievable in the home. Search **www.shopdiabetes.org** or search for portion control tools online, and you'll find plenty to choose from.

When to Weigh and Measure

It is very important to weigh and measure your foods when you begin to count carbohydrates. If you weigh and measure all your foods and beverages for a couple of weeks, you will learn a lot about the correct serving size—and you may be surprised by the size your usual portions! Don't worry; you do not have to weigh and measure foods every day forever. It's not practical or realistic to expect yourself to do so, especially when you eat away from home. The more you practice weighing and measuring foods and beverages, the easier it is to estimate correct servings when you don't have these tools available. However, you'll always want to weigh or measure new foods.

Once you're able to eyeball the correct serving size, you can estimate most of the time and occasionally weigh or measure the foods you regularly eat to check that your eyes are still seeing correct serving sizes—those portions can slowly grow over time. It's also a good idea to go back to weighing and measuring foods when you see your blood glucose levels or your weight start to climb. These numbers might be on the rise because your portions have grown.

The bottom line for mastering serving sizes is honesty. If you are honest with yourself, your servings will be on the money more times than not. Learn more tips and tricks to estimate portions when you eat away from home in Chapter 10.

Tips and Tricks for Estimating Serving Sizes

Thumb tip (from first knuckle) = **1 tsp**
  Example: 1 tsp mayonnaise or margarine

Thumb (whole—to second knuckle) = **1 Tbsp**
  Example: 1 Tbsp salad dressing or cream cheese

Two fingers lengthwise = **1 oz**
  Example: 1 oz cheese or meat

Palm of hand = **3 oz**
  Example: 3 oz boneless cooked meat
  (a regular size deck of cards or a bar of soap are also good examples)

Tight fist = **1/2 cup**
  Example: 1 serving noodles or rice, 1 serving canned fruit

Loose fist/Cupped hand = **1 cup**
  Example: 1 cup vegetables or pasta

These guidelines hold true for most women's hands, but some men's hands are much larger. Use your hands to check it out for yourself!

At home, try to serve meals in same-sized plates, glasses, and bowls. This will help you judge correct portions, and you won't have to use the measuring tools so often. Try this to practice: measure a serving in a measuring cup first and then take note of how much room 1 cup of pasta takes on a dinner plate, 1/2 cup of hot oatmeal in a bowl, or 1/2 cup of milk in a glass. Keep these "pictures" in your mind for next time. Then every so often, verify that your servings are still on target.

If you serve family-style meals—that means filling large serving bowls and putting them on the table for everyone to help themselves—stop! Serving food this way promotes overeating because second helpings are that much closer to your fork and lips. Begin to serve in the kitchen. If people want seconds, they have to walk to get them. If no one needs seconds, wrap them up before you begin to eat.

Weighing and Measuring in the Grocery Store

When you purchase fresh fruits and vegetables, take advantage of the food scales that hang in the market produce area. Weigh individual pieces of fruit. Focus on what a 4-ounce banana, 6 1/2-ounce orange, or 3 1/2-ounce kiwi really looks like. These all represent 1 carbohydrate serving or 15 grams of carbohydrate. Think about your shopping and eating habits. Do you reach for the largest apple or banana and count it as one serving (15 grams) of carbohydrate, but it's really 1 1/2 carb servings (22 grams) or even 2 carb servings (30 grams)? Buy pieces of fruit that fit your needs or realize that half a piece is closer to the serving size and grams of carbohydrate you need.

It's easy to go overboard on servings of meat, poultry, and cheese because one more ounce does not look like that much more. However, each extra ounce can add another 35–100 calories, depending on the fat content. Try this: When you buy a package of cheese, cold cuts, or anything you buy by the ounce, glance at the ounces on the label. Then visualize what one, two, or three ounces looks like. If you buy cheese or cold cuts sliced at the deli counter, think about how many meals you need to make before you place your order. Let that be your guide to how many ounces you buy. If you make a smoked turkey and Swiss cheese sandwich for lunch with 2 ounces

Raw to Cooked: Rules of Thumb

Raw meat with no bone: 4 ounces raw to get 3 ounces cooked.

Raw meat with bone: 5 ounces raw to get 3 ounces cooked.

Raw poultry with skin: 4 1/4 to 4 1/2 ounces to get 3 ounces cooked. The extra 1/4 to 1/2 ounces accounts for the skin. (Remove the skin before or after cooking.)

Here is an example for a whole chicken: Each family member needs about 3 oz cooked chicken. There are five family members. The chicken has bones and skin, so you need to estimate that you'll need about 5 1/2 ounces of raw chicken per person. So, 5 × 5 1/2 = 28 ounces or about 1 3/4 pounds. If you want enough for two meals, you need about 3 1/2 pounds. Do not forget a few ounces for the organs stuffed in the cavity. So, you need about a 4-pound raw chicken.

of turkey and 1 ounce of cheese, how many sandwiches are you going to make until the next time you shop? Buy just the amount you need. The same goes for buying meat. Think about how many people you are feeding, what quantity you will lose in cooking (see *Raw to Cooked: Rules of Thumb* on page 54), and how much you want for leftovers. Then use this information to estimate the amount of raw meat you need to buy. Another benefit of this approach is that you will waste less food and in turn save some money.

Meet Rita

Rita is 52 years old and was diagnosed with type 2 diabetes about a year ago. She has struggled with her weight for years. Her nurse practitioner put her on a blood glucose–lowering medication that initially helped lower her blood glucose levels, but eventually, she put on another 12 pounds rather than losing weight. She was frustrated and didn't feel like she could get her blood glucose under control. The nurse practitioner suggested she see a dietitian, who encouraged her to keep a food diary records for two weeks before her next appointment. The dietitian also asked Rita to bring her meter and blood glucose monitoring records to her visit.

While reviewing her records, the dietitian noted that Rita just wrote down the types of foods she ate, but not the amounts. Rita generally made healthy food choices, and she explained that she didn't think it was necessary to weigh the foods if she was making healthy choices and watching her fat intake. The dietitian pointed out that because Rita has to count her calories to lose some weight, she would do better if she weighed and measured her foods as often as possible. She also taught Rita the principles of basic carb counting and encouraged her to choose three servings of carbohydrate at breakfast, four at lunch, and four at dinner. When Rita saw the serving sizes of the food models, she was amazed at how small the portions looked. The dietitian urged Rita to get a food scale and to use it in addition to the measuring cups and spoons she already had at home.

Rita went back to see the dietitian four weeks later with complete records in hand. She was pleased because she lost 1 1/2 pounds, and her blood glucose results had inched down as well. Rita said that once she started weighing and measuring her foods, she realized how much she had been eating before. She believes she can continue to lose weight if she continues to be honest about how much she eats. The dietitian suggested that Rita add some physical activity to her schedule to help her burn calories and lower her blood glucose. Rita set a goal of doing more gardening and taking a 15-minute walk two to three evenings a week.

At her next appointment two months later, Rita had lost four more pounds and her A1C had decreased from 8.2% to 7.4%. Rita and her diabetes care providers were thrilled with the results of her efforts.

6

◆◆◆◆◆◆◆◆◆◆◆◆◆◆◆◆◆◆◆◆◆◆◆◆◆◆◆◆◆◆◆◆

The Food Label Has the Facts

Today, supermarkets are nutrient data warehouses! Why? Because of the Nutrition Facts label on most foods. The Nutrition Facts label is one of the most complete sources for the nutrient content of foods. And it's free! There's no charge for reading the fine print or for comparing the numbers on several different labels.

As a carb counter, you'll find that the listing for Total Carbohydrate in the Nutrition Facts is worth its weight in gold.

In This Chapter, You'll Learn:

What information is on the Nutrition Facts label

How to use nutrition information to count carbohydrate

How to use sugar-free foods and low-calorie sweeteners or sugar substitutes

What's On the Nutrition Facts Label?

To become better acquainted with the Nutrition Facts label, it will be helpful to go through the information that it provides.

NUTRITION FACTS

Manufacturers are required by law to provide Nutrition Facts information in this easy-to-read format. The information tells you the serving size and the servings per container, as well as the calories, calories from fat, and grams of total fat, saturated fat, sodium, total carbohydrate, dietary fiber, sugars, protein, and selected vitamins and minerals in one serving of the food.

Serving Size—All of the nutrition information on the label is based on one serving, not the whole package or container, unless it is a single-serving container. Serving sizes for categories of food are set by the U.S. Food and Drug Administration (FDA), so serving sizes are consistent among different manufacturers. For example, one serving of most types of dry cereal is 3/4 cup. Serving sizes are also listed both in common household amounts (such as 4 crackers or 3/4 cup of pasta) as well as metric measures (for example, 28 grams).

Nutrition Facts

Serving Size 1 cup (228g)
Servings Per Container 2

Amount Per Serving

Calories 260   **Calories from Fat** 120

	% Daily Value*
Total Fat 13g	**20%**
Saturated Fat 5g	**25%**
Trans Fat 2g	
Cholesterol 30mg	**10%**
Sodium 660mg	**28%**
Total Carbohydrate 31g	**10%**
Dietary Fiber 0g	**0%**
Sugars 5g	
Protein 5g	

Vitamin A 4%	•	Vitamin C 2%
Calcium 15%	•	Iron 4%

*Percent Daily Values are based on a 2,000 calorie diet. Your Daily Values may be higher or lower depending on your calorie needs.

	Calories:	2,000	2,500
Total Fat	Less than	65g	80g
Sat Fat	Less than	20g	25g
Cholesterol	Less than	300mg	300mg
Sodium	Less than	2,400mg	2,400mg
Total Carbohydrate		300g	375g
Dietary Fiber		25g	30g

Calories per gram:
Fat 9   •   Carbohydrate 4   •   Protein 4

Servings per Container—This is the number of servings in the container.

Calories—This is the number of calories in one serving, listed in bold print.

Calories from Fat—Manufacturers get this number from multiplying the number of grams of fat by nine, because there are 9 calories in 1 gram of fat.

Total Fat—The total grams of fat in the serving are listed in bold print.

Saturated Fat—The grams of saturated fat are listed under Total Fat, indented, and not in bold print. Saturated fat is part of the total fat.

Trans Fat—Due to concerns about trans fat and heart disease, the FDA now requires food manufacturers to include the number of grams of trans fats in their products on the Nutrition Facts label.

Polyunsaturated Fat and Monounsaturated Fat—These are listed under Total Fat, indented, and not in bold print. These types of fat are listed voluntarily by the manufacturer or if the manufacturer makes a nutrition claim about them.

Cholesterol—The milligrams of cholesterol are listed per serving in bold print.

Sodium—The milligrams of sodium are listed per serving in bold print.

Total Carbohydrate—All of the grams of carbohydrate in one serving are listed in bold print. This is the number that you should review when you count carbohydrate. Below Total Carbs and indented in lighter print are Dietary Fiber and Sugars.

Dietary Fiber—The grams of dietary fiber per serving are listed under Total Carbohydrate and indented because fiber is part of the total carbohydrate.

Fiber Claims on the Food Label

Fiber Claim	Means
High or excellent source per serving	5 grams or more of fiber
Good source	2.5–4.9 grams per serving
More, enriched, or added	At least 2.5 grams per serving

Sugars—The grams of sugars per serving are listed under Total Carbohydrate and indented because sugars are part of the carbohydrate in the food. Many people with diabetes focus only on the sugars. There is no need to do this! When you read the Nutrition Facts, look at the grams of Total Carbohydrate first. You don't need to single out the grams of sugars. When you count the carbohydrates, you have already counted the sugars.

These sugars can be natural sugars, such as the lactose in milk or the sucrose in fruit, or added sugars, such as corn sweeteners, high-fructose corn syrup, fruit juice, molasses, agave nectar, and brown sugar. There is no way to tell from the Nutrition Facts label whether the sources are naturally occurring or added. Instead, check the ingredient list for the sources of added sugars. If the added sugars start to stack up, it tells you something about how nutritious—or not—the food is.

Protein—The grams of protein per serving are in bold print.

Vitamins and Minerals—Unlike the other information on the Nutrition Facts label, vitamins and minerals are not presented as a straightforward measured quantity (like, for example, 8 grams of fat). Instead, they are presented as percentages of a Recommended Daily Intake (RDI). (You may be familiar with the term Recommended Daily Allowance or RDA; RDI is the new term.) There are different RDI levels for different vitamins and minerals. The food label must list the percentage of the RDI for two vitamins—A and C—and two minerals—calcium and iron. Other vitamins and minerals are required to be listed if the manufacturer makes claims about them. They can also be listed voluntarily. For example, if a food is fortified with folic acid, the Nutrition Facts must state the amount of folic acid per serving.

Remember, all of the nutrition information on the Nutrition Facts label is based on one serving. Use the serving sizes on the label to help you learn what reasonable portions are. If you usually eat a larger quantity of that food, perhaps your portions are too large or the portion you may be counting as one serving is actually two or three.

It is important to point out that the food label serving size is not necessarily the same as a serving for carb counting. When it comes to foods that contain carbohydrate, remember the number 15. If you are counting carbohydrate servings, one carb serving consists of a food that has about 15 grams of carbohydrate.

For example, if you were to look at the Nutrition Facts label for a cold cereal, you may see that it says a 1-cup serving has 49 grams of carbohydrate. When you divide 49 by 15, you see that this serving size is actually three carb servings, with 4 grams of carbohydrate left over. So, a serving of 1 cup of this cereal is a little over three carb servings. If you are counting carbohydrate by grams, check the serving size and grams of total carbohydrate on the label and make sure your serving size is the same or adjust your carb count for the size of the serving you eat.

Nutrition Claims

SUGAR-FREE, NO-SUGAR-ADDED: WHAT'S THE LOWDOWN?

Foods labeled "sugar-free" or "no-sugar-added" aren't necessarily free of carbohydrate or calories. How much or little carbohydrate they contain depends on what sweeteners are in the food. Ingredients such as sorbitol and mannitol contain carbohydrate and calories. Others, such as aspartame and sucralose, don't contain calories or carbohydrate. To count carbohydrate effectively, you must know how to recognize which sweeteners contain carbohydrate and/or calories and, if necessary, account for them.

Nonnutritive sweeteners (sugar substitutes)

There are currently six nonnutritive sweeteners approved by the FDA: acesulfame-potassium, aspartame, neotame, saccharin, sucralose, and stevia (or rebiana). These are used in many foods and beverages today, including diet sodas, fruit drinks, syrups, and yogurts. The sweeteners contain no calories or carbohydrate and can greatly lower the carbohydrate and calories in foods. They don't, on their own, cause a rise in blood glucose levels. The foods they are used to sweeten may or may not contain carbohydrate and calories from other ingredients. For example, consider a diet soda with no calories versus a yogurt that contains some calories and carbohydrate from other ingredients.

Polyols

Polyols, or sugar alcohols, are another type of sweetener used in sugar-free foods. They contain, on average, half the calories of sugars (2 calories vs. 4 calories per gram); however, some have as few as 0.2 calories per gram and others are as high as 3 calories per gram. Polyols are often used in foods such as candy, cookies, snack bars, and ice creams. Look for the "-ol" ending to identify a polyol; common ones are sorbitol, lactitol, maltitol, and mannitol.

Polyols aren't completely digested by the body—that's why they have about half the calories of sugar. For the same reason, polyols can cause a lower rise in blood glucose than regular sugars. (In large amounts and in some people, sugar alcohols may cause gas, cramps, and/or diarrhea. Foods with certain amounts of polyols are required by the FDA to have a label about this possible "laxative effect.")

Some foods may contain more than one type of sweetener. Read ingredient lists carefully to find out what sweeteners are used; by law, they must all be listed. For example, Truvia, a stevia product on the market, contains rebiana, the compound in the stevia leaf that makes it sweet, in addition to erythritol, which is a sugar alcohol.

How to count sugar-free foods

Often, when people are first diagnosed with diabetes, they think they won't be able to eat sweets anymore. In this situation, some people seek out the "sugar-free" or "no-sugar-added" foods in the supermarket.

It's up to you whether you include these foods in your eating plan. If you enjoy sweets, sugar-free products can help you satisfy that craving without adding to your carb count or your waistline. But as you're learning, it's also possible to fit foods sweetened with regular sweeteners into your eating plan, as long as it is in moderation. The choice is up to you.

If you choose to eat sugar-free foods, you'll need to learn how to include these foods in your carb counts.

NET CARB, IMPACT CARB, ETC.

Some of these terms became commonplace when low-carb weight loss plans like The Atkins Diet were all the rage. Although these terms aren't as common as they once were, food manufacturers may still use these terms and others to promote their products to people watching their carbohydrate intake. To arrive at "net carbs," the manufacturers subtract the total grams of sugar alcohols and fiber from the grams of Total Carbohydrate in the product. The remaining grams of carbohydrate are then referred to as "net carbs." Some manufacturers also include a statement that only the net carbs in the product have an impact on blood glucose. It is important to know that these terms are not approved or regulated by the FDA and that the ADA does not use the term.

OTHER NUTRITION CLAIMS

Food manufacturers can make other claims on the food label outside of the Nutrition Facts label, such as "calorie-free" or "sugar-free." But what do these claims mean? Food labeling laws include rules for these kinds of claims. For an explanation of what they mean, see Table 6-1.

Table 6-1 Nutrition Claims on the Food Label

Nutrition claim	Meaning
Calorie free	Less than 5 calories per serving
Fat free	Less than 0.5 grams of fat per serving
Sugar free	Less than 0.5 grams of sugars per serving
Reduced calorie	At least 25% fewer calories than regular food
Reduced fat	At least 25% less fat than regular food
Reduced sugars	At least 25% less sugar than regular food
No added sugar, without added sugar, no sugar added	Permitted if no amount of sugars or ingredient that substitutes for sugar is used, contains no fruit juice concentrate or jelly, and the label says the food is not low calorie

Try Your Hand at Using Food Labels

It will be important for you to be able to use the Nutrition Facts label to successfully count carbohydrate. Use these samples for practice.

1. For breakfast, you have cooked oat bran cereal. The Nutrition Facts label says 1 serving is 1/3 cup and 1 serving contains 19 grams of carbohydrate and 5 grams of fiber. You eat 2/3 cup as a serving. The serving size of 2/3 cup cooked oat bran contains 38 grams carbohydrate (19 grams + 19 grams). Then you add 1/2 cup milk (6 grams carbohydrate) and 1 tablespoon raisins (7 grams carbohydrate), for a total of 51 grams carbohydrate (38 grams + 6 grams + 7 grams). If you are counting carb servings, this comes out to 3 1/2 carb servings (51 grams ÷ 15 grams carbohydrate per carb serving = 3.5 carb servings).

2. For dinner you decide to eat a frozen entrée of manicotti, a salad, a roll, and yogurt and strawberries for dessert. You read the Total Carbohydrate on the Nutrition Facts label for the prepared foods, and you get the carbohydrate counts for the roll, salad, and strawberries from a book or online database. What's your total carb intake for the whole meal?

Item	Carbohydrate (g)
Three-cheese manicotti frozen entrée	41
1 dinner roll	19
1 cup salad greens	7
2 Tbsp fat-free Catalina dressing	11
1 1/4 cup sliced strawberries	15
1/2 cup orange frozen yogurt	26
Total carbohydrate	119

If you use carb servings, how many servings would this meal add up to?
119 grams of carbohydrate ÷ 15 grams of carbohydrate per carb serving = 8 carb servings

3. For breakfast, you eat dry cereal. You mix three cereals together to get a bunch of fiber and a unique taste. You also add 2 Tbsp of raisins. What's the total carbohydrate count for this breakfast?

Item	Your Cereal (grams of carbohydrate)	Nutrition Facts (grams of carbohydrate)
1/2 cup Bran Flakes	12	24 grams in 1 cup (3 grams fiber)
1/2 cup Shredded Wheat 'n Bran	23	47 grams in 1 cup (5 grams fiber)
1/3 cup low-fat Granola	24	48 grams in 2/3 cup (2 grams fiber)
2 Tbsp raisins	15	15 grams in 2 Tbsp (2 grams fiber)
1 cup fat-free milk	12	12
Total carb count	86	

Your servings of the three cereals are half of the serving sizes listed on the Nutrition Facts labels. You also need to add the carbohydrate for the raisins and milk, too.

How many carb servings are in this breakfast?
86 ÷ 15 = 5 1/2 carb servings

7

◆◆◆◆◆◆◆◆◆◆◆◆◆◆◆◆◆◆◆◆◆◆◆◆◆◆

Carb Counting in Real Life:
How to Count Convenience Foods and Recipes

Some days, you need all the help you can get to put together a meal for yourself and your family. On those days, ready-to-eat and pre-prepped foods can be a big help. Other days, you may enjoy cooking from scratch or trying a new recipe you've clipped out of a magazine.

Both of these approaches to cooking can be accommodated by carb counting. Your eating style does not have to change because of carb counting; in fact, when you become skilled at carb counting, you may enjoy using convenience foods or some of your old recipes even

In This Chapter, You'll Learn:

How to count convenience and ready-to-eat foods

How to calculate the carb count of your favorite recipes

About resources that can help you plan carb-counting–friendly meals

more because you'll be able to predict how the meal will affect your blood glucose level.

Convenience and Ready-to-Eat Foods

The convenience foods category includes everything from a frozen pizza to a prepared entrée from the supermarket deli counter. When you count carbs, some convenience foods can actually be a blessing because they give you the carb count right on the Nutrition

Facts label. However, some ready-to-eat foods don't come with a label, like supermarket deli items and fresh baked goods.

In some cases, you can get the information you need by doing a little research. But in many cases, you'll have to use your guesstimating skills. You'll learn how in this chapter.

The How To's

Let's start with some frozen convenience foods you might buy in the supermarket. Here's the Nutrition Facts for a frozen cheese pizza:

Nutrition Facts

Serving Size 1/3 pizza (120g)
Servings Per Container 3

Amount Per Serving

Calories 320   **Calories from Fat** 117

% Daily Value**

Total Fat 13g	**20%**
Saturated Fat 6g	**30%**
Trans Fat 0g	
Cholesterol 30mg	**10%**
Sodium 870mg	**36%**
Total Carbohydrate 35g	**12%**
Dietary Fiber 2g	**8%**
Sugars 7g	
Protein 14g	**28%**

**Percent Daily Values are based on a 2,000 calorie diet. Your Daily Values may be higher or lower depending on your calorie needs.

	Calories:	2,000	2,500
Total Fat	Less than	65g	80g
Sat Fat	Less than	20g	25g
Cholesterol	Less than	300mg	300mg
Sodium	Less than	2,400mg	2,400mg
Potassium		3,500mg	3,500mg
Total Carbohydrate		300g	375g
Dietary Fiber		25g	30g

Calories per gram:
Fat 9 • Carbohydrate 4 • Protein 4

If you eat one serving—or 1/3 of the pizza—you'll get 35 grams of carbohydrate, or about two carb servings. If you eat half of the pizza, what would the carb count be?

If the whole pizza (35 grams of carbohydrate per serving × 3 servings for a whole pizza) contains 105 grams of carbohydrate, then 1/2 of the pizza contains 53 grams of carbohydrate (105 ÷ 2) or 3 1/2 carb servings (53 ÷ 15).

How about a frozen lean entrée? Here's the nutrition information for a Salisbury steak with mashed potatoes and green beans:

Nutrition Facts

Serving Size 1 (269g)
Servings Per Container 1

Amount Per Serving

Calories 260   **Calories from Fat** 81

	% Daily Value**
Total Fat 9g	**14%**
Saturated Fat 4.5g	**23%**
Trans Fat 0g	
Cholesterol 45mg	**15%**
Sodium 660mg	**28%**
Total Carbohydrate 24g	**8%**
Dietary Fiber 3g	**12%**
Sugars 4g	
Protein 24g	**48%**

**Percent Daily Values are based on a 2,000 calorie diet. Your Daily Values may be higher or lower depending on your calorie needs.

	Calories:	2,000	2,500
Total Fat	Less than	65g	80g
Sat Fat	Less than	20g	25g
Cholesterol	Less than	300mg	300mg
Sodium	Less than	2,400mg	2,400mg
Potassium		3,500mg	3,500mg
Total Carbohydrate		300g	375g
Dietary Fiber		25g	30g

Calories per gram:
Fat 9 • Carbohydrate 4 • Protein 4

So, the complete entrée has 24 grams of carbohydrate or about 1 1/2 carb servings. You might add a salad, a cup of soup, and/or a dinner roll. Add it all up and you've got your carb count.

How about a canned soup? Here's lentil soup with vegetables:

Nutrition Facts

Serving Size 1 cup (250g)
Servings Per Container About 3

Amount Per Serving

Calories 170   **Calories from Fat** 14

% Daily Value**

Total Fat 1.5g	**2%**
Saturated Fat 0g	**0%**
Trans Fat 0g	
Cholesterol 0mg	**0%**
Sodium 710mg	**30%**
Total Carbohydrate 30g	**10%**
Dietary Fiber 7g	**28%**
Sugars 2g	
Protein 10g	**20%**

**Percent Daily Values are based on a 2,000 calorie diet. Your Daily Values may be higher or lower depending on your calorie needs.

	Calories:	2,000	2,500
Total Fat	Less than	65g	80g
Sat Fat	Less than	20g	25g
Cholesterol	Less than	300mg	300mg
Sodium	Less than	2,400mg	2,400mg
Potassium		3,500mg	3,500mg
Total Carbohydrate		300g	375g
Dietary Fiber		25g	30g

Calories per gram:
Fat 9   •   Carbohydrate 4   •   Protein 4

If you have 1 cup of soup—or 1/3 of the can—you'll get 30 grams of carbohydrate, or about 2 carb servings. Next, add up the carbohydrate from the other items in your meal for your total carb count.

These examples are fairly easy because you have the nutrition information right in front of you. Just be sure that you calculate the carbohydrate based on the amount you actually eat and not the serving size on the label.

It gets tougher when you don't have a Nutrition Facts label. Let's look at an example. Let's assume you get a bagel with cream cheese on your way to work in the morning. You look at the carb count for a bagel in Appendix 1 and note that half of a 1-ounce (oz) bagel (which is a small bagel) has 15 grams of carbohydrate. You know the bagels that you buy are pretty large, but you're not sure how much they weigh.

So, how do you find nutrition information for these types of foods? You have a couple of choices. On a supermarket trip you can see if you find any bagels that are the size of the ones you get. If they are packaged, they will have a Nutrition Facts label, or you can try asking at the bakery for nutrition information. Check out the weight of these bagels, estimate how close or far they are from the ones you purchase, and do the math from there. A second approach is to calculate an average from a variety of sources. Appendix 2 includes some references for restaurant foods. Look up bagels and take an average of the amount of carbohydrate listed for the different sources. You can also check restaurant websites, and add their information into your calculation. With all this information—and of course your honesty about portion size—you'll likely be very close. Then record the information in your personal database (see Chapter 3), so you'll have the information readily available next time.

Here's an example of how this might play out. This is the nutrition information for a bagel found packaged in the supermarket:

Nutrition Facts

Serving Size 1 (103g)
Servings Per Container 6

Amount Per Serving

Calories 264   **Calories from Fat** 14

	% Daily Value**
Total Fat 1.5g	**2%**
Saturated Fat 0g	**0%**
Trans Fat 0g	
Cholesterol 0mg	**0%**
Sodium 427mg	**18%**
Total Carbohydrate 53g	**18%**
Dietary Fiber 2g	**8%**
Sugars 10g	
Protein 11g	**22%**

**Percent Daily Values are based on a 2,000 calorie diet. Your Daily Values may be higher or lower depending on your calorie needs.

	Calories:	2,000	2,500
Total Fat	Less than	65g	80g
Sat Fat	Less than	20g	25g
Cholesterol	Less than	300mg	300mg
Sodium	Less than	2,400mg	2,400mg
Potassium		3,500mg	3,500mg
Total Carbohydrate		300g	375g
Dietary Fiber		25g	30g

Calories per gram:
Fat 9   •   Carbohydrate 4   •   Protein 4

From this information you know this bagel weighs about 3 1/2 ounces (103 grams ÷ 30 grams in an ounce = 3.5). Each bagel contains 53 grams of carbohydrate or 3 1/2 carb servings. You eyeball it and determine that it's a bit smaller than the one you buy at the coffee shop.

Next you check out bagels on the Dunkin' Donuts website. You note that their plain bagel is closer to the size of the bagel you buy. There is no weight on it, but you look at the nutrition information.

Nutrition Facts

Serving Size 1
Servings Per Container

Amount Per Serving

Calories 260   **Calories from Fat** 27

	% Daily Value**
Total Fat 3g	**5%**
Saturated Fat 0.5g	**3%**
Trans Fat 0g	
Cholesterol 0mg	**0%**
Sodium 780mg	**33%**
Total Carbohydrate 69g	**23%**
Dietary Fiber 2g	**8%**
Sugars 6g	
Protein 14g	**28%**

**Percent Daily Values are based on a 2,000 calorie diet. Your Daily Values may be higher or lower depending on your calorie needs.

		Calories: 2,000	2,500
Total Fat	Less than	65g	80g
Sat Fat	Less than	20g	25g
Cholesterol	Less than	300mg	300mg
Sodium	Less than	2,400mg	2,400mg
Potassium		3,500mg	3,500mg
Total Carbohydrate		300g	375g
Dietary Fiber		25g	30g

Calories per gram:
Fat 9   •   Carbohydrate 4   •   Protein 4

You notice that this bagel contains 69 grams of carbohydrate, or 4 1/2 carb servings. Now, to factor in the cream cheese. You see that one packet of cream cheese only adds 3 grams of carbohydrate. It does, however, add another 130 calories!

As you go through this process, you might find that you eat more carbohydrate and calories than you thought you did. To correct that, you may consider eating only half of the bagel at breakfast.

Try this again, this time with some items you might pick up at the deli counter. Maybe you regularly buy prepared coleslaw (the light vinegar-based type) and baked beans for quick weeknight side dishes. Now you're wondering about their carb counts, but they don't come with a Nutrition Facts label. One day you ask the deli clerk for their nutrition information. You find that the Nutrition Facts on the coleslaw are:

Nutrition Facts

Serving Size 1/2 cup
Servings Per Container

Amount Per Serving

Calories 41   **Calories from Fat** 14

                                                 % Daily Value**

Total Fat 1.5g	**3%**
Saturated Fat 0g	**0%**
Trans Fat 0g	
Cholesterol 0mg	**0%**
Sodium 14mg	**1%**
Total Carbohydrate 8g	**3%**
Dietary Fiber 1g	**4%**
Sugars 3g	
Protein 1g	**2%**

**Percent Daily Values are based on a 2,000 calorie diet. Your Daily Values may be higher or lower depending on your calorie needs.

	Calories:	2,000	2,500
Total Fat	Less than	65g	80g
Sat Fat	Less than	20g	25g
Cholesterol	Less than	300mg	300mg
Sodium	Less than	2,400mg	2,400mg
Potassium		3,500mg	3,500mg
Total Carbohydrate		300g	375g
Dietary Fiber		25g	30g

Calories per gram:
Fat 9   •   Carbohydrate 4   •   Protein 4

This is a pleasant surprise. It turns out this coleslaw is an easy way to eat an extra serving or two of vegetables without taking in too many calories.

You find that the Nutrition Facts for the barbecued baked beans are:

Nutrition Facts

Serving Size 1/2 cup
Servings Per Container

Amount Per Serving

Calories 180   **Calories from Fat** 36

	% Daily Value**
Total Fat 4g	**6%**
Saturated Fat 1g	**5%**
Trans Fat 0g	
Cholesterol 0mg	**0%**
Sodium 360mg	**15%**
Total Carbohydrate 32g	**11%**
Dietary Fiber 8g	**32%**
Sugars 14g	
Protein 5g	**10%**

**Percent Daily Values are based on a 2,000 calorie diet. Your Daily Values may be higher or lower depending on your calorie needs.

	Calories:	2,000	2,500
Total Fat	Less than	65g	80g
Sat Fat	Less than	20g	25g
Cholesterol	Less than	300mg	300mg
Sodium	Less than	2,400mg	2,400mg
Potassium		3,500mg	3,500mg
Total Carbohydrate		300g	375g
Dietary Fiber		25g	30g

Calories per gram:
Fat 9   •   Carbohydrate 4   •   Protein 4

You know when you eat these, your serving size is closer to 3/4 cup, so you are probably getting about 48 grams of carbohydrate. Be sure to add of all this new information to your personal database. No need to go through that exercise every time you eat these foods.

Meet George

Because of his work schedule, George ate breakfast at 6 a.m. and lunch at 11:30 a.m. Between meals, around 9 a.m., he bought a cookie from the vending machine. It was called a Monster Cookie, and when he checked the Total Carbohydrate on the food label, he found it contained 35 grams. When he checked his blood glucose before lunch (which was two hours after eating the cookie), his blood glucose was in the 220–250 mg/dl range. This happened three days in a row. He didn't know why his blood glucose was running high, so he called his dietitian. She asked him to e-mail her a copy of the cookie label. She found that the serving size on the Nutrition Facts label was one cookie, though there were two cookies in the package. George reported that he ate both of them, meaning that his morning snack contained 70 grams of carbohydrate. He and his dietitian discussed a plan for better control: eat one of the cookies instead of both or replace the cookie with healthier snack, such as a piece of fresh fruit.

Your Recipes—Counting Carbs

Don't discard your favorite recipes or think that your days of clipping recipes from the newspaper or searching for them online are over. Just as you learned to estimate the nutrition information in prepared foods, you can also learn how to calculate the carbohydrate in servings from recipes.

Of course, you can avoid this exercise by using recipe books and cooking magazines that provide nutrition information. All of the American Diabetes Association's (ADA) cookbooks provide this information. In addition, most of the cookbooks and cooking magazines that are geared toward people with diabetes, people who want to lose weight, and those who are interested in healthier eating also provide carb counts for the recipes. This is a good way to get new recipes as well as learn about lower-calorie and lower-fat cooking techniques.

THE HOW-TO'S OF RECIPE CARB COUNTING

Step #1: Start by writing down each of the ingredients in the recipe and the amount used in the recipe.

Step #2: Find the grams of carbohydrate that are in the amount of each food in the recipe, use the Appendices in this book as your starting reference.

Step #3: Add up the total grams of carbohydrate from all ingredients in the whole recipe.

Step #4: Divide the total carbohydrate by the number of servings to calculate the grams of carbohydrate in one serving.

Step #5: Write this information down on the recipe and/or if it is a recipe you make regularly, write it down in your database of carb counts.

PRACTICE WITH A RECIPE

Here's an example of how you can calculate a recipe's carbohydrate content. This is the ingredient list from a recipe for Moroccan chicken stew.

Amount/Ingredients	Carbohydrate (grams)
2 cups chicken broth	0
1/4 cup tomato paste	6
1 tsp ground cumin	0
1 tsp salt	0
1/4 tsp ground red pepper	0
1/8 tsp cinnamon	0
1/2 cup dark raisins	58
1 medium-size onion, sliced thin	16
1 Tbsp minced fresh garlic	4
2 lb butternut squash	52
2 cups frozen green peas	40
1 can (16 ounces) chickpeas	108
4 chicken thighs	0
Total grams of carbohydrate	284

This recipe yields four servings. So, each serving contains 71 grams of carbohydrate (284 ÷ 4) or about five carb servings.

As with anything else, practice will increase your comfort level with this process. Select one of your favorite recipes and try to calculate the grams of carbohydrate in each serving.

ONLINE RESOURCES

The ADA website now features a tool called MyFoodAdvisor that can help you estimate the carbohydrate, calories, and other nutrients in recipes and individual food items. It allows you to save favorite recipes, as well as track the foods you eat day to day. Check it out at **www.diabetes.org**.

ADA'S MONTH OF MEALS DIABETES MEAL PLANNER

Wouldn't it be nice to plan your meals in an instant and know how many calories, carbohydrate, and fat were in each meal? That's exactly what the *ADA's Month of Meals Diabetes Meal Planner* does for you. This book is perfect for anyone who uses basic carb counting or is looking to simplify his or her meal planning with healthy, easy-to-fix recipes. The book has over 500 meals and hundreds of recipes, allowing you to make nearly endless combinations of breakfast, lunch, and dinner. Each meal tells you the nutrition facts for that specific meal, too. You can easily arrange your meals so that the carbohydrate, calorie, and fat counts will fall within your target ranges for the day. This book takes so much of the legwork out of carb counting, and we highly recommend it for anyone trying to learn how to count carbs.

8

❖ ❖

Carb Counting in Real Life:
How to Count Restaurant Meals and Take-Out Food

The average American eats four or more restaurant meals each week. Most of us have hectic, busy lives, and eating out can be convenient and fun. If restaurant meals are part of the way you eat, this doesn't have to change with carb counting. With a little practice, you can learn to apply the principles of carb counting to just about any menu item at any restaurant.

In This Chapter, You'll Learn:

How to figure the carb counts of restaurant meals

Tips to deal with large restaurant portions

How to do a "food lab" on your favorite restaurant meals

Information for the Asking

Today, there's more nutrition information available for restaurant foods than ever before. Fast food restaurants like McDonald's, Burger King, and KFC post nutritional information in their restaurants and on their websites. Some national chains like Applebee's, Pizza Hut, and Panera Bread often include nutritional information on their websites. Some also offer brochures or binders with nutrition information by request. If you often eat at these types of places, take a few minutes to visit their websites and look up the menu items you tend to order. Add this information to your personal database so you can access it easily next time.

Many smaller, independent restaurants do not generally have nutrition information readily available. This is true of fancy, special occasion restaurants as well as the mom-and-pop takeout place on the corner. When you eat in these types of restaurants, you'll need to do a little more work.

Table 8-1 Sample Personal Database Record— Restaurant Meals

Meal	Serving (amount I eat)	Grams of Carbohydrate
Restaurant: Burger King		
Original Whopper Jr. (no mayo)	1	32
French fries	1/2 medium	23
Side garden salad	1	5
Salad dressing, Catalina	2 Tbsp	5
	Total	65
Restaurant: Pizza (from local pizza parlor)[1]		
Cheese pizza with onions and mushrooms	3 slices	96
	Total	96
Restaurant: Mexican (from local Mexican restaurant)[2]		
Fajitas with	3	
Chicken and beef	4 ounces	0
Grilled onions and peppers	2/3 cup	11
Tortillas, 6 inch	3	54
Guacamole	3 Tbsp	4
Tomatoes	1/2 cup	3
Rice, Mexican	1/3 cup	16
Refried beans	1/2 cup	20
	Total	108

[1]Estimate based on an average of nutrition information from Pizza Hut, Domino's, and Papa John's from the *ADA Guide to Healthy Restaurant Eating*, 4th edition (American Diabetes Association, 2009.
[2]Based on Nutrition Facts labels and Nutrition Information obtained from www.ars.usda.gov/nutrientdata (the USDA searchable database).

If you eat out at the same places regularly, start by writing down what you usually eat at different meals. Then estimate the size of the serving and the amount of carbohydrate in it, using the list in Appendix 1 and the resources listed in Appendix 2. If you have records of your blood glucose levels after eating these meals, put that down, too. These records will provide clues about how well you are estimating the carbohydrate in your restaurant meals. Be sure to include the beverages you drink, whether they are carbonated, fruit juices, alcoholic, or calorie-free. Some of these beverages have carbohydrates and calories, and you may not realize how much you are consuming.

Tips to Make Your Best Guess

If you weigh and measure foods regularly at home, you'll be familiar with portion sizes. Remember to use these skills in restaurants, too. Measuring portions by comparing them to your hands and common household items (see the list in Chapter 5, on page 53) can be particularly helpful in restaurants, where you don't have access to measuring spoons, cups or a food scale.

If there's no nutrition information for the restaurant, look for the same or similar dish on the website of a national chain; use this information as a starting point for your estimation. For example, the nutrition information for chicken parmesan listed on the Macaroni Grill website can help you estimate the carb count in the chicken parmesan you get at your favorite local Italian place. To get even more accurate, check out the carb counts for the same dish at several different places and take an average.

If you're a regular and you have a few items you regularly order, the restaurant staff may be willing to share a recipe with you so you can estimate the carb count based on the techniques we covered in the last chapter.

Another helpful tactic is to order your favorite dishes for take-out, so you can weigh and measure the portions at home. You can weigh the pieces of meat and bread, measure the servings of rice or pasta, and estimate the content of sauces and coatings. This exercise is usually quite eye-opening—restaurant portions are often quite large! You may realize that one meal should become two.

If you can't find information on some foods you regularly eat, see if you can find a recipe for a similar dish on a recipe website, in a cookbook in the library, or in the collection of a friend of family member. Then use the recipe analysis techniques covered in Chapter 7. Don't forget sauces! They often contain added sugar, flour, or corn starch, all of which contain carbohydrate and impact blood glucose.

Restaurant Eating: Tips and Skills

One of the biggest problems with restaurant meals is that the portions are huge. Here are tips and tactics to help you control your portions and thus, carbs and calories:

- Avoid items on the menu that include words like large, giant, grande, supreme, extra large, jumbo, double, triple, double-decker, king-size, monster, and super. Instead, choose items described as junior, single, petite, kiddie, and regular.
- If you see a weight for a piece of meat on the menu, it's most likely the raw weight. For example, you might see a hamburger referred to as a "quarter pound" of meat, a fillet weighing 6 ounces, or a slice of prime rib that weighs 10 ounces. Remember that these are averages—not exact weights. Refer to *Raw to Cooked: Rules of Thumb* on page 54 to help you convert servings from raw weight to cooked weight.
- Consider ordering soup and salad, or an appetizer and a salad or soup. That may be enough for you.
- Ask for a half portion or share an entrée with another person.
- Ask for a takeout container at the beginning of the meal, and place the extra food in it to take home.

A NOTE ABOUT PIZZA

Pizza can be challenging for some people with diabetes. It can cause blood glucose to rise in some people, and it can cause a delayed rise in blood glucose in other people. For starters, when you eat pizza, do your best to get a solid carb count. Use some of the techniques described in the book: check the websites of national chains and take an average of the carb counts you find for similar types of pizza.

Then check your blood glucose two hours after you eat. If there is a lot of meat and cheese on the pizza and/or if your two-hour blood glucose wasn't what you expected, check your blood glucose again three to five hours after starting the meal. If your blood glucose is high, then the high fat content in the pizza could have been the cause. Keep close records the next time you eat pizza, too. This is important information to know—and you'll use it every time you eat pizza.

A Closer Look—Lunch at a Restaurant

It's easy to lose track of your carbohydrate targets when you're eating out. Menu choices that seem "light" can often have lots of hidden carbohydrate. Let's say you go out to lunch and have soup and salad. That sounds like a good choice—but it all depends on what you put on your salad and what type of soup you have.

Food	Carbohydrate (g)
3 cups salad greens	8
bacon bits, egg, ham	0
1/3 cup kidney beans	15
1/3 cup chickpeas	15
1 cup croutons	15
1/3 cup fat-free salad dressing	15
1 1/2 cups chicken noodle soup	30
Total carbohydrate	98, or 6 1/2 carb servings

This so-called "light" lunch can easily put you way above your target. How can you bring down the carb count of this meal?
- Reduce the amount of croutons to 1/2 cup and save 8 grams of carbohydrate.
- Reduce the salad dressing to 1 Tbsp and save 12 grams of carbohydrate.
- Combine the kidney and chickpeas in a 1/3 cup serving and save 15 grams of carbohydrate.
- Add 1 cup of a combination of broccoli, cauliflower, and carrots for 5 grams of carbohydrate.
- Only have 1 cup of the soup and save 10 grams of carbohydrate.

With these changes, your total savings is 45 grams of carbohydrate, and you're back in range without giving up too much flavor or quantity of food.

Meet JB

JB worked at the mall, and ate all his lunches at the food court during the workweek. He rotated his choices from the various ethnic cafes and generally ordered the same item each time. He was trying to eat 60–75 grams of carbohydrate at lunch, but his records showed that sometimes his blood glucose levels were too high after lunch. So his dietitian suggested that they do a "food lab" with his food choices. He bought one of each of his usual lunch choices for takeout. Together JB and his dietitian measured the carbohydrate in each.

Here's what they found:

Lunch #1: Vegetable stir-fry with fried rice. This meal dishes up 2 1/2 cups of fried rice, which has 105 grams of carbohydrate. The stir-fry veggies were all nonstarchy vegetables, such as broccoli and bok choy, and there were 1 1/2 cups of them, or 15 grams of carbohydrate. Chinese food (and some other ethnic cuisines) can also contain hidden carbohydrate that comes from sugar in marinades and sauces and from the cornstarch used to thicken sauces. A handy guidline is to add 5–10 grams of carbohydrate to your total to account for this hidden carbohydrate. All told, this meal had 120 grams of carbohydrate, which was nearly twice as much as the 60- to 75-gram target range. When he checked his blood glucose level after the meal, it was 235 mg/dl. This showed that the larger amount of carbohydrate raised his blood glucose higher than he wanted it to be two hours after the meal.

Lunch #2: Two small beef enchiladas. They figured that this meal had 35 grams of carbohydrate—much less than his target level. When he checked his blood glucose level two hours later, it was 60 mg/dl, and he had to treat a low blood glucose level (hypoglycemia). He needed to add either a serving of Mexican rice or refried beans to his lunch to get more carbohydrate in the meal.

Lunch #3: A gyro sandwich with cucumber salad. The sandwich had thick pita bread as the wrap, and it was filled with lean lamb. The pita bread weighed 2 ounces, so it counted as 30 grams of carbohydrate. The cucumber salad was 1 cup of cucumbers and 1/3 cup of yogurt, equal to 5 grams of carbohydrate. The lamb had no carbohydrate. So the total for the meal was 35 grams of carbohydrate, much below his target of 60–75 grams. They checked his blood glucose log, and it showed a glucose level of 65 mg/dl after the meal. JB needed to add a medium-sized piece of fruit and a glass of milk to add 30 grams of carbohydrate to the meal and bring the total up to 65 grams of carbohydrate in the meal.

Lunch #4: Sushi and miso soup. The rice in the sushi was the source of the carbohydrate in the meal. Fortunately, JB really likes sushi, so he ate enough rolls to reach his target of 60 grams of carbohydrate.

Lunch #5: Two slices of deep-dish pizza with sausage and extra cheese with a small garden salad and Thousand Island dressing. They estimated that each large slice of the pizza had 37 grams of carbohydrate, and he was eating two large slices. With a total of 74 grams of carbohydrate in the pizza alone, his blood glucose level two hours later was 185 mg/dl—higher than he wanted. He planned to order two medium-size pieces of the pizza in the future. The dietitian suggested that thin-crust pizza is lower in carbohydrate, especially with only a regular amount of cheese and some nonstarchy veggies, such as mushrooms, peppers, and onions.

9

◆ ◆

Blood Glucose Pattern Management:
Fine-Tuning Your Control

You've learned how to identify carbohydrate in the foods you eat, how to add it all up, and how to track your blood glucose levels. You've even learned how to record other things that can play a role in blood glucose control, such as exercise and stress. Now what do you do with all this information?

The next step is what diabetes health care providers call "pattern management." Pattern management is a way to use your records to learn how your body reacts to a variety of factors and then adjust your diabetes plan and your daily activities to get the best possible blood glucose control.

> **In This Chapter, You'll Learn:**
>
> About pattern management and how it can help you
>
> How technology can help with pattern management
>
> About the role record keeping plays in pattern management

Keep in mind, for most people with diabetes, there is no such thing as "perfect" control. But you certainly can minimize the ups and downs—and keeping your blood glucose levels in your target zones most of the time is the best way to keep yourself healthy today and for years to come.

It isn't possible to keep blood glucose in perfect control all the time because blood glucose results are affected by more than just the carbohydrate you eat. Blood glucose levels depend on what your blood glucose level was before you ate, the stress you're under, your physical activity (yesterday and today), your level of insulin resistance all the time and at different times of the day, how much protein and fat you've eaten, how fast or slowly you ate, and on and on and on.

Remember you are a unique individual, and every time you sit down to eat, it is a new physical-chemical-emotional interaction. The only way to get a handle on the many factors that can affect your blood glucose is to build your own "database of experiences." This is how pattern management works, and why your records are so important. Learning from your own experiences will help you control your diabetes more than anything else. Eventually, you'll be able to predict how your body will react in most of the usual daily situations.

Pattern Management: It Takes Three Steps

In Chapter 3, we covered the information you should include in your daily log. Appendix 3 is a sample log sheet that you can use or adapt to your needs. Now, we'll work with that information to identify and interpret the patterns.

STEP 1. FIND THE PATTERNS

You will need:
- A few weeks' worth of blood glucose records that contain at least two blood glucose checks each day
- Two color markers or highlighters—one color for high levels (above your target), one color for low levels (below 70 mg/dl)
- Your blood glucose targets. Talk with your health care providers about your target blood glucose levels. In general, ideal blood glucose target ranges are:
  - Before meals: 70–130 mg/dl
  - After meals (one to two hours after start): less than 180 mg/dl

Go through your records and mark any blood glucose readings that are above your target with one color. Mark any low readings with the other color.

STEP 2. OBSERVE THE PATTERNS

Now look for patterns in your highs and lows. If many of your blood glucose results are above your target range, consider whether one or several of the following could be the cause:

- Not taking the correct dose of medication, needing an increased dose, or needing additional or different medications (take your records and observations to your provider)
- Too much carbohydrate at the meal
- Less physical activity than planned
- Physical or emotional stress
- A high-protein and/or high-fat meal

If many of your blood glucose values are below the target range, consider whether one or several of the following could be the cause:

- Delayed or missed meals or snacks
- Too little carbohydrate at meals or snacks
- Not taking the correct dose of blood glucose–lowering medication that can cause hypoglycemia or needing a dose adjustment

STEP 3. PLAN AND TAKE ACTION

After you've identified patterns, plan a course of action to limit these situations in the future. Sometimes a simple change, like adjusting your eating plan, is enough. For example, you may have found that a couple of hours after dinner, your blood glucose is usually higher than your target. Your records reveal that you've been eating more carbohydrate than you should at dinner. Therefore, a logical action would be to eat the amount of carbohydrate you should be eating, then check your blood glucose a few evenings to determine whether this change has brought your blood glucose levels into your target range.

If your blood glucose results are consistently above 250 mg/dl or below 70 mg/dl, don't wait—contact or make an appointment with your diabetes care provider to get help adjusting your diabetes plan. More than likely, you need adjustments in your blood glucose–lowering medication.

Trouble Finding Patterns?

What do you do when there is a variation in your blood glucose levels but no specific pattern? Look for changes in your daily schedule, such as missed meals or differing amounts of physical activity. When you check your records, do you find:

Missed meals or snacks?	❏ yes	❏ no
Variable activity?	❏ yes	❏ no
Stress?	❏ yes	❏ no
Varied eating schedule?	❏ yes	❏ no
Different amount of carbs?	❏ yes	❏ no

If you answered "yes" to several or all of these, then do you also find in your records:

Insulin doses that change often?	❏ yes	❏ no
Frequent hypoglycemia?	❏ yes	❏ no
Frequent hyperglycemia?	❏ yes	❏ no

There is a connection between the changes in the first list and the results in the second list. Usually, the problem reveals itself in your records, and it can be fixed with a few small adjustments. You may be miscalculating the grams of carbohydrate in your meals, or you may need to do more precise measuring for a while to get your portions back on track. There is no substitute for blood glucose checks and keeping detailed records to sort out the changes in patterns. Discuss the changes and possible causes and solutions with your health care provider. You can also refer to Chapter 11 for more information on using advanced carb counting to adjust insulin doses.

Is There Data Management Technology for Pattern Management?

Yes. Today, most blood glucose monitors double as data management systems, allowing you to save your blood glucose results in the device's memory. The results can then be downloaded to your personal computer with the assistance of software provided by or purchased from the monitor's manufacturer.

Each monitor's data management software works a little differently and offers different features. Some models can be integrated with a PDA (personal digital assistant) or a smartphone. Some include carb counting and/or calorie counting databases.

Today there are even continuous glucose monitors (CGMs) that can provide glucose readings around the clock. These monitors remain attached to your body through a sensor—a fine needle with an attached small transmitter—that stays under your skin, much like the way an insulin pump is attached. Depending on the model and the programming (only three are approved by the FDA to date), CGMs will capture a glucose reading anywhere from every five minutes to every hour. Some CGMs can store up to seven days' worth of results, which can then be downloaded into a data management system on your computer.

To learn what's available with various blood glucose monitors and CGM devices, visit the manufacturers' websites. Technology is evolving rapidly, and new functionalities are introduced frequently.

Time for Real-Life Practice

Let's look at how pattern management works with some practical examples. Here are two examples of how pattern management can help a person with diabetes gain better control.

Meet FW

FW is newly diagnosed with type 2 diabetes and was just started on a low starting dose of 500 mg of metformin. He is 45 years old. He is 5'10" tall and weighs 225 pounds. His target blood glucose range for fasting and before meals is 70–130 mg/dl and for two hours after meals is less than 180 mg/dl. He wanted to give carb counting a try, so he kept a log of two meals for a day to see how much carbohydrate he was eating and the effect it had on his blood glucose levels. He did not have target carbohydrate goals because he did not know how much he was eating at meals. His record of two meals on one day is on pages 94–95.

Step 1. Find the Patterns

FW went through his two days of records and highlighted his high and low blood glucose levels with colored markers.

Step 2. Observe the Patterns

Then he was able to see a pattern. He started his day with a high blood glucose reading. His breakfast and lunch carbohydrate grams were between 124 and 139, which was too high and was causing the high after-meal blood glucose levels. He did no physical activity before or after those meals to help bring the high blood glucose levels down. He now understood why he had symptoms of high blood glucose, such as being thirsty and having to urinate a lot.

Step 3. Plan and Take Action

This information helped him make some decisions. FW decided to take a 15-minute walk after lunch. He discussed the amount of carbohydrate he should eat at his meals with a dietitian. He said he was willing to cut down some and shoot for a range of 80–90 grams of carbohydrate per meal. Then he would keep records for three days (a weekend day and two workdays) and go through the three-step process again to see if he needed to make further adjustments.

Meet Roberta

Roberta is 60 years old, lives alone, and has type 2 diabetes. She had learned carbohydrate counting and was keeping records to see if she could achieve her target blood glucose goals. She has a target blood glucose goal, fasting and before meals, of 120 mg/dl, and a two-hour after-meal blood glucose target of 190 mg/dl. She takes a combination of two blood glucose–lowering medications, pioglitazone and glimepiride, in one pill (Actos; see her medication record on pages 94–95). She was keeping this record to see how much carbohydrate she was eating, how it affected her blood glucose level, and whether her physical activity and medication had a positive effect on her blood glucose levels.

Step 1. Find the Patterns

Roberta checked for blood glucose levels that were in or out of range. Her fasting, after breakfast, before lunch, after lunch, before dinner, and after dinner were all out of range.

Step 2. Observe the Patterns

She looked for patterns. She found that she ate too much carbohydrate at breakfast. Over 100 grams was simply too much. She was delighted to see that a 30-minute walk before dinner helped keep the after-meal blood glucose lower than it was after lunch with the same amount of carbohydrate. However, it was still too high. She also noticed that her fasting blood glucose was high—160–180 mg/dl, on average.

Step 3. Plan and Take Action

She decided to cut her breakfast down to 1/2 cup of oatmeal, use low-fat milk (which saves calories, but not carbohydrate), and add 1/2 banana. That would cut her carbohydrate to about 75 grams. She also planned to eat smaller portions at lunch and dinner, keeping the carb count to between 65 and 75 grams.

This is a middle step, as these are still high amounts for a small lady like Roberta. She was willing to keep logs for a few days with these changes and see what effect they had on her blood glucose levels. Because Roberta is not taking the maximum dose for her blood glucose–lowering medication and she has had type 2 diabetes for about eight years, it might be that she needs more or different medications. She will discuss her records and observations with her health care provider at her upcoming visit.

FW's Carb Counting and Blood Glucose Record

Day/Date: Monday

Time/meal	Diabetes medicines		Food		
	Type	Amount	Type	Amount	Carb grams
8:30 a/ breakfast	None		Sausage	2	0
			Biscuit, 2 oz	1	34
			Banana, med.	1	30
			Orange juice (fast food)	16 oz.	60
					Total 124
2:00 p/ lunch			Cheeseburgers, Jr.	2	68
			Fries	small	33
			Chocolate chip cookies (fast food)	3	38
					Total 139

Notes about day:

Roberta's Carb Counting and Blood Glucose Record

Day/Date: Monday

Time/meal	Diabetes medicines		Food		
	Type	Amount	Type	Amount	Carb grams
8:00 a/ breakfast	Piogli- tazone/ glimepi- ride	30 mg/ 2 mg	Oatmeal, 1 pkg.	1 cup	68
			Whole milk	1 cup	12
			Banana, large	1	25
					Total 105
12:30 p/ lunch			Macaroni & cheese	2 cups	54
			Apple juice	1 cup	30
					Total 84
6:30 p / dinner			Soup, chicken noodle, Campbell's	2 cups	30
			Crackers, saltine	12	12
			Canned fruit cocktail, water packed	1 cup	22
					Total 64

Notes about day:

Blood glucose results							
Fasting/ before b'fast/ time	After b'fast/ time	Before lunch/ time	After lunch/ time	Before dinner/ time	After dinner/ time	Before bed/ time	Other/ time
240/ 7:35 a	308/ 10:00 a						
		228/ 1:45 p	318/ 3:45 p				

Blood glucose results							
Fasting/ before b'fast/ time	After b'fast/ time	Before lunch/ time	After lunch/ time	Before dinner/ time	After dinner/ time	Before bed/ time	Other/ time
174/ 7:30 a	208/ 10:15 a						
		196/ 12:15 p	280/ 1:45 p				
				180/ 6:15 p	216/ 7:50 p		30 minute walk before dinner

Don't Check Lots, Check Smart

Hopefully these sample records have helped you understand the value of record keeping and pattern management. Each person will check his or her blood glucose levels on different schedules; the frequency depends on your needs and desires, whether you have recently made an adjustment in your regimen, and whether you regularly adjust your medication based on your results. Depending on your situation and the type of medication you take, you may check your blood glucose two to three times a day a few times a week, or upwards of six times a day every day. Another option is to use a CGM device intermittently to check the effect of carbohydrate on glucose levels. No matter how often you check, keep in mind that you want to check smart versus a lot. Checking smart means checking strategically. Always have in mind why and what you are checking and what information this check will provide. Yes, blood glucose monitoring and record keeping is an investment of time and energy, but it can pay big dividends in day-to-day and long-term health.

10

◆◆◆◆◆◆◆◆◆◆◆◆◆◆◆◆◆◆◆◆◆◆◆◆◆◆◆◆◆◆◆

Blood Glucose–Lowering Medications and Insulin

Today, there are a variety of categories of medications available to help lower blood glucose. Each category of medicines works in different ways. All people with type 1 diabetes require insulin, whether they get it by injection or an insulin pump. Most people with type 2 diabetes need to take one or more medications. Which medications you take and how many generally depends on the number of years you've had type 2 diabetes, how well you've cared for it, and how successful you've been in making lifestyle changes. All of these medication options

In This Chapter, You'll Learn:

About different kinds of blood glucose–lowering medications

About which medications can cause hypoglycemia and how to treat it

About insulin pumps and pens

allow you and your health care providers to find the approach that most closely matches your diabetes and lifestyle needs.

If you are taking insulin, either through multiple daily injections or an insulin pump, advanced carb counting will help you calculate your insulin doses and keep your blood glucose levels on target. Chapter 11 will give you all the details on advanced carb counting; for now, here's a review all of the available medication options, how they work, and what things you need to consider when taking them.

There are two basic categories of diabetes medications: oral medications and injectable medications. These medications use different mechanisms to help lower blood glucose levels, such as increasing insulin production, reducing insulin resistance, and/or reducing glucose absorption. Insulin is injected into the body when the pancreas cannot produce any or enough insulin to control your blood glucose. People with type 1 diabetes use insulin from the time of diagnosis, and about 50–60% of people with type 2 diabetes eventually need to take insulin along with other medications to control their blood glucose levels.

Oral Medications

Oral medications include several different classes of drugs, including sulfonylureas, meglitinides, biguanides, thiazolidinediones, alpha-glucosidase inhibitors, DPP-4 inhibitors, bile acid sequestrants, and dopamine agonists. The brand names of these drugs and whether they cause hypoglycemia is shown in Table 10-1.

- **Sulfonylureas** have been around since the 1950s. They stimulate certain cells in the pancreas, called beta-cells, to release more insulin, which lowers blood glucose levels. These can only work if you still make some insulin.
- **Meglitinides** also stimulate the beta-cells in the pancreas to release more insulin.
- **Biguanides** (metformin) lower blood glucose levels by reducing the amount of glucose produced by the liver. They also make muscle tissue more sensitive to insulin, so glucose can be absorbed. Metformin, now a generic medication, is today the most commonly used starting medication for people with type 2 diabetes.
- **Thiazolidinediones** (sometimes called glitazones) reduce the amount of glucose produced by the liver and help insulin work better in muscle and fat. Recent studies have shown that this class of medication may increase the risk of heart failure and bone fractures in some people, so be sure to discuss this with your health care team if you take a thiazolidinedione.
- **Alpha-glucosidase inhibitors** slow the breakdown of starches, such as bread, potatoes, and pasta, in the intestine. This slows the rise in blood glucose levels after a meal.
- **DDP-4 inhibitors** help slow the breakdown of a naturally occurring compound in the body, called glucagon-like pep-

tide-1 (or GLP-1). GLP-1 normally lowers blood glucose levels in the body by inhibiting the release of glucagon from the pancrease, increasing the release of insulin, and slowing the speed of digestion. People with type 2 diabetes have been found to be deficient in GLP-1 and other so-called incretin hormones. DPP-4 inhibitors slow the breakdown of GLP-1. This allows it to work longer in order to complete its normal functions.

- **Bile acid sequestrants** have only recently been identified in the treatment of diabetes. Colesevelam is the only FDA-approved medication from this class. It is primarily used to lower LDL (or "bad") cholesterol, but when it is combined with a sulfonylurea regimen, it has been found to lower blood glucose levels.

Table 10-1 Oral Medications

Class of Medication	Generic Name	Brand Names	Can Cause Hypoglycemia?
Sulfonylurea	glimepiride	Amaryl	YES
	glipizide	Glucotrol, Glucotrol XL	
	glyburide	Diabeta, Glynase, Micronase	
Meglitinide	repaglinide	Prandin	YES
	nateglinide	Starlix	
Biguanide	metformin	Glucophage, Glucophage XR, Glumetza, Fortamet, Riomet (liquid)	NO
Thiazolidin-edione	pioglitazone	Actos	NO
	rosiglitazone	Avandia	
Alpha-glucosidase inhibitor	acarbose	Precose	NO
	miglitol	Glyset	
DPP-4 inhibitor	sitagliptin	Januvia	NO
	saxagliptin	Onglyza	
Bile acid sequestrants	colesevelam	Welchol	NO
Dopamine agonist	bromocriptine	Cycloset	NO

- The **dopamine agonist bromocriptine** was approved by the FDA for treatment of type 2 diabetes in 2009. An older version of this drug was used in higher doses to treat Parkinson's disease, but studies have shown that it can also be used to lower blood glucose levels.

Injectable Medications

Injectable medications include an amylin analog, incretin mimetics, and, of course, insulin, which is covered in its own section of this chapter. The brand names of these drugs and whether they cause hypoglycemia is shown in Table 10-2.

- The **amylin analog pramlintide** is a synthetic form of the hormone amylin, which is also produced in the pancreatic beta-cells and is secreted with insulin. Amylin works with insulin and glucagon (another hormone) to maintain blood glucose levels. People with diabetes are amylin deficient. Pramlintide injections have been shown to lower blood glucose levels without causing hypoglycemia or weight gain.
- Two **incretin mimetics** are approved by the FDA: **exenatide** and **liraglutide**. Incretin mimetics, also called GLP-1 analogs, stimulate insulin secretion and decrease glucagon release from the beta-cells in the pancreas. They also lower the rise of glucose after eating. With these actions, incretin mimetics decrease appetite and food intake and have shown some success in helping people lose some weight.

Table 10-2 Injectable Medications

Class of Medication	Generic Name	Brand Names	Can Cause Hypoglycemia?
Amylin analog	pramlintide	Symlin	NO
Incretin mimetic	exenatide	Byetta	NO
	liraglutide	Victoza	

Insulin

Insulin is classified by how quickly or how long it works in the body. You'll hear insulin referred to as rapid acting, short acting, intermediate acting, and long acting. This refers to how long it takes for the medicine to have an effect on blood glucose and how long the effect lasts. Note that all insulins can cause hypoglycemia. Table 10-3 shows different types of insulin and the timing of their activity. Figure 10-1 shows how those insulins fit into a daily routine with meals.

Table 10-3 The Action of Insulins

Insulin	Onset	Peak	Duration
Rapid acting			
lispro (Humalog)	~15 minutes	1–2 hours	3–5 hours
aspart (Novolog)	~15 minutes	1–2 hours	3–5 hours
glulisine (Apidra)	~15 minutes	1–2 hours	3 5 hours
Short acting			
regular	0.5–1 hour	2–3 hours	3–6 hours
Intermediate			
NPH (isophane)	2–4 hours	4–10 hours	10–16 hours
Long acting			
glargine (Lantus)	3–4 hours	8–16 hours	24 hours
detemir (Levemir)	3–4 hours	6–8 hours	14 hours

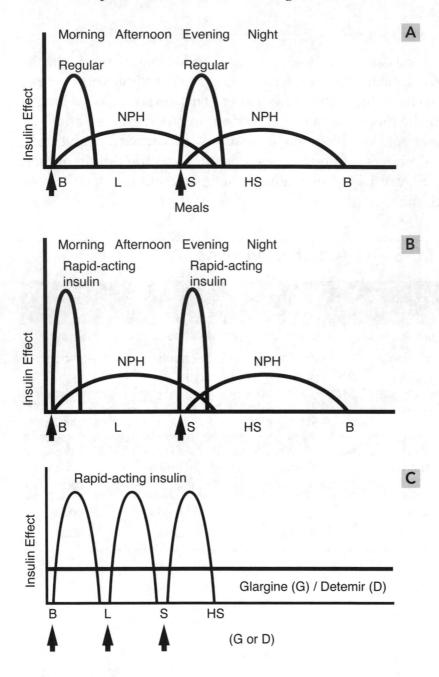

Figure 10-1
A. Short-acting and intermediate-acting insulin.
B. Rapid-acting and intermediate-acting insulin.
C. Rapid-acting insulin with meals and long-acting insulin in the evening.
Left to right:
B = breakfast, **L** = lunch, **S** = supper, **HS** = evening snack, **B** = bedtime

HOW MUCH INSULIN DO YOU NEED?

Unfortunately, there's no simple answer to this question. There are many ifs, ands, and buts. Health care providers have a variety of ways of deciding starting insulin doses. Even more, insulin needs can change as you move through different phases of your life or make changes in your routine. For example, women have different insulin needs in different phases of their menstrual cycle or in different trimesters of pregnancy. A man in retirement who gets into long-distance bicycling will have different insulin needs than he did before starting his new hobby. Adolescents during growth spurts have varying insulin needs.

Keep in mind that a starting dose of insulin is just that—a place to start. The next step is to use your records to fine-tune your insulin needs based on your blood glucose results. However, it's always best to start conservatively, whether you're just starting on insulin or moving from insulin by injection to an insulin pump. Better to be safe (and not increase the risk of hypoglycemia) than sorry.

What's the Difference Between Rapid-Acting and Short-Acting Insulin?

As you might guess, rapid-acting insulin works more quickly than short-acting insulin, which is known as regular insulin. The beauty of rapid-acting insulin is that the peak of its action is more likely to coincide with the rise in blood glucose from the food you've eaten—in about one to two hours. As the carbohydrate raises your blood glucose, the rapid-acting insulin is beginning to lower your blood glucose. Regular insulin doesn't peak until three to four hours after the meal and can miss the mark, so to speak. Experts agree that the rapid-acting insulins aren't even as rapid as people need to control after-meal blood glucose rises. Drug development is ongoing to find even faster-acting insulins. In the meantime, it's best to take the rapid-acting insulin 15 minutes prior to eating, when possible.

Know Your Medications

It is important that you know the type of blood glucose–lowering medication(s) you take, when to take each one, how they work to help control blood glucose, and how the medication works in conjunction with the carbohydrate you eat to control your blood glucose. Talk with your diabetes care providers to make sure you have all of the information you need. Be sure to record the type, dose, and timing of each medication daily. You can record it along with your blood glucose results and your food diary, or you may use another form; refer to Chapter 3 for more information on record keeping. Whatever method you choose, this information will help you and your health care providers interpret your blood glucose results.

Carb Counting, Medications, and Hypoglycemia

Carb counting and pattern management are critical to the effective use of blood glucose–lowering medications. Most medications work to lower blood glucose not to increase it. But you can get too much of a good thing! Some medications may cause blood glucose to drop too low if you don't eat enough carbohydrate or don't account for other changes in your routine. Low blood glucose levels (below 70 mg/dl) can cause headache, dizziness, disorientation, irritability, and blurred vision, and in serious cases, it can lead to unconsciousness.

Studies have shown that serious hypoglycemia is rare among people with type 2 diabetes, even if they are taking insulin or one of the oral medications that can cause it (see Tables 10-1 and 10-2). The most serious risk is for people with type 1 diabetes. However, anyone who takes a medication that can cause hypoglycemia should be aware of the condition, how to prevent it, how to recognize it, and how to treat it if it occurs.

HOW DO I KNOW IF I HAVE HYPOGLYCEMIA?

Most people experience one or more of the following symptoms of hypoglycemia:
- Shakiness
- Dizziness
- Sweating
- Hunger

- Headache
- Pale skin color
- Sudden moodiness or behavior changes, such as crying for no apparent reason
- Clumsiness or jerky movements
- Seizure
- Difficulty paying attention or confusion
- Tingling sensations around the mouth

Some people don't experience any of these symptoms. If you have any doubts, check your blood glucose level.

HOW TO TREAT HYPOGLYCEMIA

Even when you are consciously trying to prevent hypoglycemia, it can surprise you. Therefore, you need to be ready to deal with it, if it happens. If you feel that your blood glucose level is already slipping too low, treat first and then check your blood glucose level.

The **Rule of 15** is a good place to start. Eat 15 grams of carbohydrate and wait 15 minutes. Then check your blood glucose level and make sure it is on the upswing. If it is still less than 70 mg/dl, then repeat these steps.

Examples of 15 grams of carbohydrate:
- Four glucose tablets (each has 4 grams of carbohydrate)
- Glucose gel or other preparations of pure glucose
- 4–6 ounces of fruit juice (any type)
- 4–6 ounces of regular soda (not diet)
- 10–15 jellybeans

The glucose tablets and gels, as well as other pure forms of glucose, are preferred because they can raise blood glucose more quickly. Sources such as fruit juice and regular soda contain some glucose and some fructose; fructose raises blood sugar more slowly. Also, the sources of pure glucose are easy to carry with you. It's a good idea to carry some source of glucose with you at all times if you are at risk of hypoglycemia. You can carry glucose tablets in your purse, pocket, briefcase, backpack, and the glove compartment of your car. Keep them at your bedside for nighttime lows. Do be especially careful about driving if you suspect that you have hypoglycemia, especially if you have been drinking alcohol, which can cause hypoglycemia. If you think your blood glucose may be headed down, check it before you start to drive.

Once you've experienced hypoglycemia, make note of your symptoms and share them with your family, friends, and coworkers so they can recognize it. When your blood glucose goes too low, your thinking and coordination may be impaired, and in extreme cases, you can lose consciousness. It's important that family, friends, and coworkers know that you have diabetes, the signs of hypoglycemia, and what they should do for you if you can't help yourself.

WHAT CAN YOU DO TO PREVENT HYPOGLYCEMIA?

To reduce the chances you'll develop hypoglycemia, it's important to know what can cause hypoglycemia. Hypoglycemia can arise when you take a medication that causes hypoglycemia and you don't eat enough carbohydrate or enough food at a meal, miss a meal, or increase your amount of physical activity. If you are regularly experiencing low blood glucose, immediately contact your diabetes care provider. You probably need to have your medications adjusted.

To prevent lows, be sure to observe the amount of carbohydrate you are eating at meals. Try to eat your target amount of carbohydrate at regularly spaced meals. Also, it is important to take the correct dose of medicine at the proper time. If you get more physical activity than usual, you may need to eat more carbohydrate. Check your blood glucose before the activity. If your blood glucose level is 100 mg/dl or less, consider eating some carbohydrate before you exercise. This is particularly important if you will be active for more than 30 minutes. Then check your blood glucose after the activity to determine whether you need more carbohydrate. Your blood glucose is likely to decrease over the next few hours because the body uses more glucose during and after exercise.

Can I Adjust My Medication Doses on My Own?

The only blood glucose–lowering medication that you should adjust on your own is insulin. If you take any other kind of diabetes medication, oral or injectable, and you think that your dosage needs to be adjusted, then you should contact your diabetes care provider.

If you do take insulin and want to adjust doses on your own, you should ask yourself these two questions:

- How comfortable do you and your diabetes health care provider feel about you making these adjustments? If you aren't currently comfortable, what do you need to learn in order to be comfortable?
- How much time you are willing and able to take to check your blood glucose and do pattern management?

11

◆◆◆◆◆◆◆◆◆◆◆◆◆◆◆◆◆◆◆◆◆◆◆◆◆◆◆◆◆

Advanced Carb Counting

At this point, you've got some experience using basic carb counting to manage your blood glucose levels. If you take insulin, you may want or need to move on to advanced carb counting. This is used by people who use an insulin pump or take rapid-acting insulin at mealtimes along with a daily dose of longer-acting insulin to allow for insulin adjustment. If you are in one of these situations, you could gain flexibility and better control of your blood glucose levels with advanced carb counting.

In This Chapter, You'll Learn:

Whether you want or need to move on to advanced carb counting

How to calculate your insulin-to-carbohydrate ratio

How to calculate and use correction factors

With advanced carb counting, it's not necessary to eat the same amount of carbohydrate at each meal throughout the day. Instead, you adjust your pre-meal rapid-acting insulin dose to match up with the amount of carbohydrate you eat. Although this gives you greater flexibility in your eating plan, it does involve more complex tracking and calculations.

Take the self-assessment on page 110 to see if you are ready, willing, and able to move on to advanced carb counting.

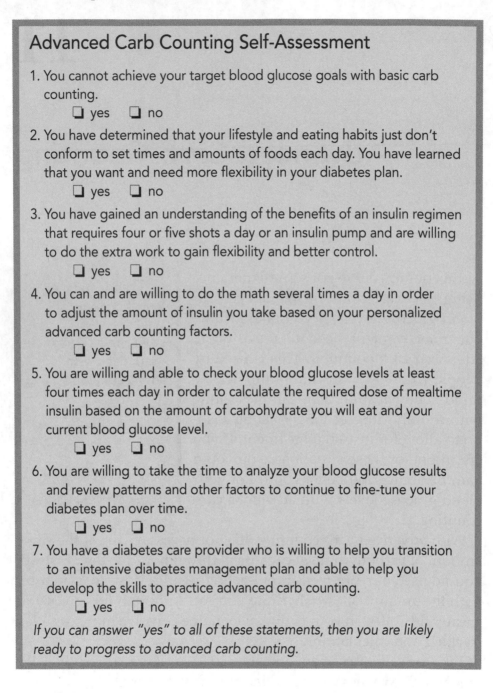

Advanced Carb Counting Self-Assessment

1. You cannot achieve your target blood glucose goals with basic carb counting.
   ❏ yes   ❏ no

2. You have determined that your lifestyle and eating habits just don't conform to set times and amounts of foods each day. You have learned that you want and need more flexibility in your diabetes plan.
   ❏ yes   ❏ no

3. You have gained an understanding of the benefits of an insulin regimen that requires four or five shots a day or an insulin pump and are willing to do the extra work to gain flexibility and better control.
   ❏ yes   ❏ no

4. You can and are willing to do the math several times a day in order to adjust the amount of insulin you take based on your personalized advanced carb counting factors.
   ❏ yes   ❏ no

5. You are willing and able to check your blood glucose levels at least four times each day in order to calculate the required dose of mealtime insulin based on the amount of carbohydrate you will eat and your current blood glucose level.
   ❏ yes   ❏ no

6. You are willing to take the time to analyze your blood glucose results and review patterns and other factors to continue to fine-tune your diabetes plan over time.
   ❏ yes   ❏ no

7. You have a diabetes care provider who is willing to help you transition to an intensive diabetes management plan and able to help you develop the skills to practice advanced carb counting.
   ❏ yes   ❏ no

If you can answer "yes" to all of these statements, then you are likely ready to progress to advanced carb counting.

Advanced Carb Counting—the Ins and Outs

Advanced carb counting is not a do-it-yourself approach. As explained earlier, advanced carb counting is usually used in conjunction with a multiple-injection insulin regimen or an insulin pump. This approach is often referred to as intensive diabetes management. If you're ready for advanced carb counting, we encourage you to work with diabetes care providers who are knowledgeable about intensive diabetes management and are willing to give you the time you need to apply these techniques.

MANAGING INSULIN ACTION

When you take rapid-acting insulin, it affects your blood glucose for 3–4 hours afterward. Therefore, your dose of insulin depends on what you predict your body will do in the future, based on what you eat, what you do, and all of the other factors we've discussed that can affect blood glucose levels. This is called "prospective management," and it's the best way to achieve blood glucose control with insulin.

Some people get caught up in a giant rollercoaster ride by managing blood glucose "retrospectively." This means treating high blood glucose levels that have already occurred with insulin that works in the future. Obviously, this doesn't work very well.

Some health care providers still teach retrospective management—for example, your health care provider may have told you to take, for example, 5 units of insulin if your blood glucose is between 150 and 200 mg/dl, 7 units of insulin if your blood glucose is between 200 and 250 mg/dl, and so on. But as noted previously, this approach doesn't work well, especially with rapid-acting insulin. For all of these reasons, we encourage you to act prospectively with advanced carb counting. The more prospective—future oriented—you can be in your estimation of your insulin needs, the better your control will be.

A New Vocabulary

To implement advanced carb counting, you'll need to master the terms below.

Basal insulin. Basal insulin is the amount of insulin you need to keep your blood glucose in control regardless of whether you eat any food. Basal insulin levels aim to mimic the normal insulin production of a healthy pancreas, about 1 unit per hour. You may also hear basal insulin referred to as "background insulin."

Insulin pumps only use rapid-acting insulin. The pump maintains a basal insulin level by pumping small amounts of insulin into the body over the entire day. The user then programs specific amounts of insulin to be released to cover the carbohydrate in meals and snacks (if eaten) and other spikes in blood glucose levels. If insulin is given by injection, a long-acting insulin is injected to cover basal needs either once or twice a day.

Over the last decade, the availability of longer-acting insulins has made basal insulin therapy easier to achieve. Today, glargine (Lantus) and detemir (Levemir) are the insulins available for basal therapy.

There are many variables to consider in figuring out your basal or background insulin dose. For example, some people's blood glucose levels go up before they wake due to a rise in hormones at that time of day (between 3 and 4 am), a situation known as the "dawn phenomenon." As a result, you may require more insulin in the morning to achieve your blood glucose targets. Some people's blood glucose levels tend to track downward in the early hours of the night, thus they need less insulin during that period. This is why it is so important to work with knowledgeable diabetes care providers to help you arrive at the correct dose.

It is also why some people choose an insulin pump. Most insulin pumps allow you to have different basal segments during the 24 hours of the day. They also allow you to have different basal rates for different days of the week—for weekday and weekend variation. These are the huge plusses of an insulin pump.

Generally, about 50% of your total insulin intake in 24 hours will be your basal insulin, but you might find you need as little as 45% (or less) or as much as 60% (or more).

Bolus insulin. When people who don't have diabetes eat, their bodies automatically release the amount of insulin they need into the bloodstream to keep blood glucose from going no higher than about 140 mg/dl. Bolus insulin is the amount of rapid-acting insulin that you need to bring your blood glucose back to pre-meal target levels within three to four hours after the start of a meal. Bolus insulin can also be used to "correct" or bring down a high blood glucose level. Bolus insulin can account for as little as 40% (or less) of the total daily insulin dose or as much as 55% (or more).

Insulin-to-carb (I:Carb) ratio. An I:Carb ratio tells you the amount of rapid-acting bolus insulin you need to bring your blood glucose level back to the pre-meal target levels within about three to four hours of starting a meal. When you use I:Carb ratios to figure your bolus insulin doses, you can be more flexible about what and how much you eat—and when you eat, too. There are different ways to calculate this ratio, depending on your circumstances. For complete details on I:Carb ratios, see "How to Determine Your I:Carb Ratio" on page 115.

Postprandial blood glucose (PPG). Postprandial blood glucose is your blood glucose level a couple of hours after you eat. It is formally defined by the American Diabetes Association (ADA) as one to two hours after the start of a meal. When you use advanced carb counting, checking your PPG is critical. It's the only way to see how well your bolus doses and I:Carb ratios are working. The ADA target for PPG is 180 mg/dl or less.

Multiple daily injection (MDI) regimen. People who take insulin and want to control their blood glucose levels closely take multiple daily insulin injections. Today this means four to five shots a day—one or two shots of a longer-acting insulin and three shots prior to mealtime.

If You're on an MDI Regimen or an Insulin Pump, Do You Need to Eat Snacks?

You can snack less often using an MDI regimen or an insulin pump, or you may be able to avoid snacks altogether, particularly if you use rapid-acting insulin. Remember that rapid-acting insulin works with the rise of blood glucose from the meal and is gone from the body within three to four hours. So, if you don't want to eat snacks, this type of plan may work well for you. If you want to eat snacks because you enjoy them or find that they help you control your blood glucose better, then you need to use blood glucose checks to determine whether you need more insulin.

How Can I Find Out More about Insulin Pumps and the Realities of Using a Pump?

Today, more and more people are choosing to go on an insulin pump. There are two types of insulin pumps available. The first type is a small device about the size of a pager. It is connected to your body by tubing or by an infusion set and cannula placed just under the skin. The device is carried in a pocket or belt holster. The other type is a tubeless system. You simply wear a pod with the insulin in it. You communicate with the pod through a pager-sized device via radio frequency. Either pump system can be programmed to provide insulin doses throughout the day. The insulin pump delivers insulin in a way that more closely mimics a normal pancreas.

Many find that an insulin pump gives them greater flexibility in managing their lives and their diabetes and that a pump helps them improve their blood glucose control. You might consider a pump if you:

• Have type 1 diabetes and want more flexibility with insulin and timing of meals
• Have type 2 diabetes and take four shots of insulin a day and want more flexibility
• Have type 1 or 2 diabetes and want better blood glucose control
• Have problems managing blood glucose levels overnight or with irregular bouts of activity

Just about anyone with diabetes, at any age, can use an insulin pump. Today most health plans cover part or all of the pump and related supplies. If you are interested in moving to a pump, talk with your diabetes care providers; if no one on your current care team is experienced with pumps, find a provider who is.

How to Determine Your I:Carb Ratio

Now that you have the advanced carb counting terms under your belt, let's move on to the two different ways you can determine your I:Carb ratio. It's best to work with your diabetes care provider to determine the best method and the best ratio for you. This section will provide a basic understanding to get you started. The first number in the I:Carb ratio represents the number of units of insulin you need to take in relation to the second number; the second number represents the number of grams of carbohydrate in the meal. So an I:Carb ratio of 1:15 means that you need to take one unit of insulin for every 15 grams of carbohydrate in the meal.

A I:Carb ratio of 1:15 is often a starting point for people new to intensive diabetes management. People who are sensitive to insulin—meaning that small amounts of insulin lower their blood glucose rapidly—might need a higher I:Carb ratio, such as 1:20. Conversely, people who are insensitive to insulin—meaning it takes a lot of insulin to lower their blood glucose—might need a lower I:Carb ratio, such as 1:10. To make things even more interesting, you might find that you need to use different I:Carb ratios at different times of the day. For example, some people who eat the same amount of carbohydrate at breakfast, lunch, and dinner need more insulin in the morning than they do at lunch or dinner, due to the "dawn phenomenon" mentioned previously.

We'll talk more about how to determine which I:Carb ratio is best for you in a minute. For now, let's work with the 1:15 ratio to give you a sense of how this method works. To calculate your I:Carb ratio this way, you'd add up the number of carbohydrate in your meal and divide that number by 15. The resulting number is the number of units of insulin you need to take. For example, let's say you're about to eat a meal that you know contains 72 grams of carbohydrate. To find out how much insulin you need to take, do the following calculation:

72 grams
÷15
4.8 (If you aren't on a pump, round up to 5)

This means you need to take 5 units of rapid-acting insulin to cover the carbohydrate in this meal.

There are two different ways to determine the right I:Carb ratio for you to use at each meal.

METHOD #1: USE YOUR FOOD DIARY AND BLOOD GLUCOSE RECORDS

Your daily records can be a valuable tool in figuring your I:Carb ratio. You'll need records for at least several days, but a whole week is even better. While you're collecting data for your I:Carb calculation, it is helpful to do blood glucose checks more often than usual—both before you eat and one to two hours after you start to eat to get your PPG. You'll also want to try to keep your carbohydrate grams and the amount of activity you do as consistent as possible day to day. This will help you establish a more precise I:Carb ratio.

Next, using the methods reviewed in Chapter 3, calculate the total grams of carbohydrate in each meal you ate. Then calculate your I:Carb ratio for each meal by dividing the total grams of carbohydrate in the meal by the number of units of rapid- or short-acting insulin you took to achieve your target blood glucose level. You might find that you get a different I:Carb ratio at different times of the day. You might also find that you need different amounts of insulin for certain foods or meals, such as pizza, a high-protein and high-fat meal, or for prolonged meals, such as a buffet dinner party.

Here's an example. Maybe you see that you generally eat about 60 grams of carbohydrate at breakfast, and you take about 4 units of rapid-acting insulin. This amount of insulin seems to get you back to your pre-meal target blood glucose within three and a half hours. That's good. To find a breakfast I:Carb ratio, you divide 60 grams of carbohydrate by 4 units of insulin. The answer is 15, or 1 unit of insulin for every 15 grams of carbohydrate—an I:Carb ratio of 1:15.

Method #1 will work if your blood glucose level is generally within your targets both before and after eating. If you are not near your targets, this method will not be as helpful because the amount of insulin you are taking is not achieving optimal blood glucose control. If this is the case, method #2 might work better as a starting point.

METHOD #2: THE GUIDELINE OF 500

As explained above, Method #2 is used for people who are having a harder time achieving control of their blood glucose levels. This method is based on two guidelines, and each can be personalized to work for you. These guidelines are based on the clinical experience and research of a number of diabetes experts who have worked with many people who use intensive diabetes management.

Method #2 uses a set number to represent the total grams of carbohydrate eaten in a day. Many clinicians use 500 as that number, especially for people who take rapid-acting insulin, which is why this method is sometimes referred to as "the guideline of 500." Some recommend using 450 instead, particularly for people who take short-acting insulin. Either way, that number is then divided by your Total Daily Dose (TDD) of insulin. To find your TDD, add up all of the units of insulin you take in 24 hours—both rapid and longer acting. Let's say your TDD is 42 units.

$$\begin{array}{r} 500 \\ \div 42 \\ \hline 12 \end{array}$$

This means your I:Carb ratio is 1:12, or 1 unit of rapid-acting insulin for every 12 grams of carbohydrate you eat in a meal or snack.

Let's say you eat a breakfast that has 60 grams of carbohydrate in it. Based on the I:Carb ratio of 1:12, how much insulin are you going to take to cover the carbohydrate in the meal? Divide the total carbohydrate in the meal by the number of grams of carbohydrate that 1 unit of insulin will cover.

$$\begin{array}{r} 60 \text{ grams} \\ \div 12 \\ \hline 5 \end{array}$$

So you will take 5 units of insulin to cover the 60 grams of carbohydrate in the meal.

COMPARE THE METHODS TO DETERMINE I:CARB RATIOS

You can see that when using Method #1, 4 units of insulin were indicated to cover a breakfast with 60 grams of carbohydrate, whereas with Method #2, 5 units of insulin were called for with the same meal. Which is right? The only answer is, it depends. The only way to check whether the I:Carb ratio works for you is to use it and check your blood glucose levels frequently. You will then use that information to adjust your personal I:Carb ratio appropriately.

Figuring Correction Factors

So far, you've learned how to calculate an insulin dose in relation to a meal. But what happens when your pre-meal blood glucose level is too high, before you even start eating? In these situations, you may need some additional insulin to get your blood glucose levels on target.

To account for this, you'll need to calculate your correction factor. The correction factor tells you how much additional rapid-acting insulin you need to get your blood glucose back to your pre-meal target level. Your correction factor depends on how sensitive you are to insulin.

This is where Method #2's second guideline comes in. This is a method for calculating correction factors, or how much 1 unit of rapid-acting insulin lowers your blood glucose.

Here's how it works. As with the guideline of 500, you need to use your TDD of insulin. Then you divide 1,800 by your TDD to determine your correction factor.

Here's an example. Let's say your TDD is 35.

$$\begin{array}{r} 1,800 \\ \underline{\div 35} \\ 51 \text{ (to simplify things, round it to 50)} \end{array}$$

This means that 1 unit of rapid-acting insulin lowers your blood glucose by 50 mg/dl. And that means that your correction factor is 1 to 50, or 1:50. (If you take short-acting insulin, your diabetes care provider may recommend using the number 1,500 instead of 1,800 for better accuracy.)

Now that you have a correction factor, try to figure out a hypothetical correction dose. Let's say you check your blood glucose before dinner, and it is 225 mg/dl. Your target pre-meal blood glucose level is 110 mg/dl. To find out how much you need to lower your blood glucose to get to your target, you subtract the target level from the actual blood glucose.

> 225 (actual blood glucose)
> –110
> ――――
> 125 (the difference between where you are
>   and where you want to be)

Now you use your correction factor to figure out how many units of insulin you need to take to lower your blood glucose by 125 mg/dl. If your correction factor is 1:50, you'd do the following calculation:

> 125
> ÷50
> ――――
> 2.5 units of insulin

So you need to take 2 1/2 units of insulin to get your blood glucose to target levels. If you take insulin by injection or with an insulin pen that counts in whole numbers, round down to 2. If you use a pump, you can take the exact dose.

If your pre-meal target is a range of 90–130 mg/dl, then you need to select one specific number within that range to use in the calculation. You may want to choose a number in the middle, either 110 or 120 mg/dl.

USING THE CORRECTION FACTOR TO FIGURE YOUR INSULIN DOSE

Using the amounts in the previous examples, you have found that you need 5 units of insulin to cover 60 grams of carbohydrate in your breakfast. You also need 2 units of insulin to bring your blood glucose back to your pre-meal target. So, to figure how much rapid-acting insulin to take, you add the two results together:

> 5 units for the meal
> +2 units to correct pre-meal levels
> ――――
> 7 units of insulin

Practice Calculating an Insulin Dose

Try to figure out a dose using the following information:

• Pre-meal blood glucose is 175 mg/dl
• Target pre-meal blood glucose is 120 mg/dl
• Correction factor is 1 unit to lower blood glucose 70 mg/dl
• Amount of carbohydrate in meal is 69 grams
• I:Carb ratio is 1:16

First, we'll figure out how much insulin you need to lower the blood glucose level.

$$\begin{array}{r} 175 \text{ (actual blood glucose)} \\ \underline{-120} \text{ (target pre-meal blood glucose)} \\ 55 \text{ mg/dl} \end{array}$$

Using the correction factor, we need to figure out how much insulin is needed to get levels into target range.

$$\begin{array}{r} 55 \text{ (actual blood glucose)} \\ \underline{\div 70} \text{ (the correction factor)} \\ 0.8 \text{ unit of insulin (round up to 1 if you don't} \\ \text{use an insulin pump)} \end{array}$$

It will take 1 unit of insulin to correct the pre-meal glucose level. Now figure out how much insulin to use to cover the carbohydrate in the meal. The I:Carb ratio is 1:16.

$$\begin{array}{r} 69 \text{ grams of carbohydrate} \\ \underline{\div 16} \\ 4.3 \text{ units of insulin (round down to 4 units} \\ \text{if you don't use an insulin pump)} \end{array}$$

Now you add the correction insulin to the meal insulin.

$$\begin{array}{r} 1 \text{ unit} \\ \underline{+4 \text{ units}} \\ 5 \text{ units} \end{array}$$

There you go! It should take 5 units of pre-meal bolus insulin to cover the meal.

It's important to look at the patterns of your blood glucose. If day after day you have to use one or more units of insulin to correct your blood glucose level before a meal, then you either need more basal insulin in the time leading up to that meal or you need to increase the bolus insulin for the previous meal. Use the information you gain to make finer adjustments to your insulin doses and stay within your target ranges all day long.

How Often Should You Change Your Correction Factor and I:Carb Ratio?

You should recalculate your correction factor and I:Carb ratio whenever your TDD moves up or down by 5 units. Many things can affect your TDD, such as becoming more active or changing the type of insulin you take. Whatever the reason, if your TDD changes, go back through the calculations. Also, examine your blood glucose records to see if you can track what's happening.

How Can You Keep Track of These Factors?

Keep a record of your current correction factor and I:Carb ratio in something that is always with you: a piece of paper in your wallet or your smartphone, for example. This way, if you forget, you know where to look. When you make a change, update these notations.

When to Take Mealtime Insulin

In a simpler world, you'd always take just enough insulin about 15 minutes before each meal to cover the exact amount of carbohydrate in that meal. Doing this will result in the best management of blood glucose levels possible. However, as we all know, this is not always possible. Here are some quick tips about taking mealtime insulin.

BE PROACTIVE

It's easier to maintain your blood glucose levels in the target range if you provide enough insulin before a meal rather than treating high blood glucose levels after the fact. So take the time to carefully calculate how many grams of carbohydrate you think you will be eating and adjust your insulin dose for that amount.

TREAT HIGH BLOOD GLUCOSE BEFORE THE MEAL

If your blood glucose is high before a meal, try to take the insulin first and then wait to see if your blood glucose levels fall before eating. To do this, you may need to check your blood glucose

30–45 minutes before a meal, take your insulin, and possibly delay eating while you wait for your levels to drop. There are a few things to note if you use this tactic for managing high blood glucose levels.

1. If you delay your mealtime insulin, the entire time of action of your insulin is delayed, which means that you may have to delay your next dose of insulin or at least consider that it is still working when it is time for your next meal.
2. DO NOT skip meals to manage high blood glucose levels. This is not a healthy choice. You may eat less at a meal or delay or skip a meal if your blood glucose levels are high once in a while. But if you are consistently high, you need to change something in your diabetes care plan—meet with your health care provider to do this.
3. Be sure to carry a carbohydrate source at all times, just in case your blood glucose gets too low and you need to treat hypoglycemia.
4. If you drive, operate machinery, or do anything else in which hypoglycemia can be dangerous to you or to others, then this treatment tactic may not be best suited for you.

PRE-MEAL HYPOGLYCEMIA

If your blood glucose is too low before a meal (less than 70 mg/dl), you have three options:

1. **Take less insulin.** This is the preferred option, especially if you are watching your weight and very conscious of the number of calories you eat. Use your correction factor in reverse, meaning that you use the correction factor to figure out how much want your blood glucose levels to rise rather than drop. For example, if your correction factor is 30 mg/dl per unit of insulin, your blood glucose level is 60 mg/dl before a meal, and your target is 90 mg/dl, then you can subtract one unit of insulin from your mealtime dose. Instead of taking insulin 15 minutes before the meal, start eating first and then take your insulin a few minutes into the meal.
2. **Eat more carbohydrate at the meal.** You could add another 15 grams of carbohydrate to the meal but not take any more

insulin. The extra 15 grams would work to raise blood glucose.

3. **Have a snack that contains 15 grams of carbohydrate before the meal.**

What you definitely don't want to do is skip or delay the mealtime insulin dose. Once the carbohydrate you eat starts to enter your bloodstream, your blood glucose will rise and you will need insulin to cover that increase in levels. With experimentation you will learn whether one way works better for you than another. In these situations, be alert for signs of hypoglycemia and treat it as soon as you sense it coming on. If you frequently have low pre-meal blood glucose levels, then you need to check your basal dose, too. Work with your diabetes care providers to make the needed adjustments to get your numbers closer to target.

UNCERTAIN CARBOHYDRATE INTAKE

If you're not sure how much carbohydrate you're going to eat at a meal, you may want to consider splitting your insulin dose. Take enough insulin 15 minutes before you eat to cover an amount of carbohydrate that you're sure you're going to eat. Then, during the meal, take the remainder of your dose to cover the remaining amount of carbohydrate in the meal. This technique works especially well if you're eating a large meal because larger-than-normal meals can cause slower rises in blood glucose levels. This is also helpful if you're eating a longer meal, like at a lengthy dinner party or a cocktail party. In situations like these, it may be better to test your blood glucose before eating the rest of the meal to help you calculate your insulin dose.

Don't Forget About "Insulin on Board"

If you are on an MDI regimen or are on an insulin pump, you'll want to pay careful attention to the amount of insulin that you still have "on board" from the last bolus dose before you determine your next bolus dose. Unfortunately, this is a concept that is often overlooked and one that, if not addressed, can lead to hypoglycemia. Keep in mind that this is not a problem for everyone; it is most common in people who react more slowly (in excess of four hours) to rapid-acting insulin.

Here's an example. Let's say you take a lunchtime bolus dose of rapid-acting insulin. Then three hours later, you have a snack with 35 grams of carbohydrate. You check your blood glucose, and it is 195 mg/dl. You want to see that blood glucose come down to your pre-meal target of 120 mg/dl. So you calculate that you need 2 units of insulin, and you need another 2 units to cover the carbohydrate in the snack. You take 4 units of insulin, and several hours later your blood glucose is 55 mg/dl. Why? Because you "stacked your insulin." You didn't consider that there was still at least one hour of action left in your lunchtime bolus dose, so you had "unused insulin" or "insulin on board."

There are several ways to avoid this. The quick and easy way is to use a higher number, such as 180 mg/dl, as your pre-meal blood glucose target when you want to take additional insulin before the action on your previous bolus insulin is complete. In the example above, this approach would have eliminated the extra 2 units.

You can also use this strategy if your blood glucose is still high a few hours after a meal and you want to get it down before you eat your next meal. For example, if it is two hours after dinner and your blood glucose is higher than you want it to be, use 180 mg/dl as your target to calculate a correction dose, rather than 120 mg/dl.

There are some helpful resources that can help you account for "insulin on board." One good source of information is John Walsh's book, *Pumping Insulin,* and his website **www.diabetesnet.com**. Both include a table that shows insulin activity at one, two, three, and four hours after bolus doses of insulin. Also, the current generation of insulin pumps has a built-in feature that helps you consider your previous bolus dose. If you ask the pump to provide your next bolus dose before the last one has been used up, the pump will ask if you want to subtract the amount of insulin still "on board" from the amount you asked it to provide. Yet another advantage of using an insulin pump! Do be aware that all of the pumps calculate insulin on board a little differently.

By now you are probably more comfortable with advanced carb counting, but even after lots of practice there will be times that you find your I:Carb ratio is not quite right and your blood glucose levels are higher than your target ranges. What can you do about it? Always start with the basics. Measure your serving sizes and the amount of carbohydrate in them. Check how well you are weighing and measuring your foods. See if your portions have grown or shrunk. Review your label reading and interpretation skills and check those for accuracy. Go through your checklist of things in your life that could have changed—your weight, your activity level, your diabetes and other medications. Doing these quick "quality assurance" checks every so often is helpful. Balancing your food, medication, and physical activity to control your blood glucose is and will remain a daily challenge. But hopefully with all this new knowledge and these skills, managing diabetes will seem like less guesswork.

Cornerstones

Knowledge and Support

You will build your diabetes knowledge base one experience at a time. But that doesn't mean you have to do it alone. In fact, you'll likely be more successful at managing your diabetes if you build a team of people around you who can provide additional knowledge and support.

For example, health care providers can offer education, insights, and resources. Family members and friends can support you and celebrate your progress. You'll find that all of these people will be valuable additions to your diabetes management team.

In This Chapter, You'll Learn:

About sources of support for your diabetes care

How to build or find a local or online support group

How to stay motivated to care for your diabetes over the years

Find Your Carb Counting Coach

If you decide carb counting is for you, a registered dietitian (RD) who is also a certified diabetes educator (CDE) can be a valuable addition to your team. An RD, CDE can be a big help in mastering basic and advanced carb counting. You can find RD, CDEs through online directories, professional associations, and local education classes. Here are some places to start:

American Diabetes Association (ADA)-recognized Diabetes Education Programs

The American Diabetes Association (ADA) has a process for recognizing diabetes education programs that meet certain quality guidelines. One of those guidelines is that a registered dietitian is part of the program (and it is likely that the RD will also be a CDE). These programs are located all over the U.S. and usually offer diabetes education group classes and one-on-one counseling. Some programs may also have exercise physiologists, pharmacists, or behavioral counselors. To find an ADA diabetes education program in your area:

- Go to the ADA website at **http://www.diabetes.org/findaprogram** and enter your zip code.
- Call the ADA at 1-800-DIABETES (1-800-342-2383). Ask for the program nearest you.

American Association of Diabetes Educators

AADE is an association of over 12,000 health professionals who provide diabetes education. To obtain the Certified Diabetes Educator (CDE) credential, an individual must go through specialized training and testing. Some diabetes care providers may take it one step further and become Board Certified in Advanced Diabetes Management (BC-ADM). To find a Certified Diabetes Educator (CDE):

- Go to **www.diabeteseducator.org/ProfessionalResources/accred/ Programs.html** to see a list of accredited programs in your area.

Do You Know the Questions to Ask?

Once you have the names of a few CDEs in your area, call and ask them a few questions about their approach to carb counting. You want to make sure you get what you are looking for. Tell them you want to learn either basic or advanced carb counting and why.

- Ask if they teach carb counting and what types.
- Ask about their experience.
- Ask how many sessions they think it will take for you to master carb counting.

- Ask if they provide their teaching only in groups or in groups and individually.
- Ask about the cost of a session or the program.
- Ask whether their services are likely to be covered by your health plan.
- Ask whether they bill your health plan or if you must submit the claim to your health care plan.

Is Diabetes Education and/or Nutrition Counseling Covered by Health Insurance?

There's no single answer to this question. The answer depends on your health coverage and the state or federal regulations that govern it. Medicare now covers diabetes education (often called diabetes self-management education [DSME] or diabetes self-management training [DSMT]) and nutrition counseling for diabetes (also referred to as medical nutrition therapy or MNT). Most states have laws requiring some health plans to cover these services as well. However, it's best to contact your health plan to get the details on coverage of diabetes education and MNT. Ask about whether the service is covered, the number of visits covered, whether you have to go to a particular person or program, and whether you need a referral for the service from your diabetes care provider.

If your health plan isn't willing to cover diabetes self-management training and/or MNT or you have no health insurance, you have to decide if you are willing and able to pay for these services. You may come to realize that a few sessions with a knowledgeable diabetes educator is not that expensive when compared to the costs of medications, hospitalizations, and even restaurant meals.

Form Your Cheerleading Squad

Beyond the how-to skills and knowledge, you need continuing support to manage the day-to-day challenges of diabetes. There will be times that you are gung-ho and feel your carb counting efforts are paying off and other times when nothing you do seems to work. Yes, you need diabetes educators to help you become more knowledgeable, but you also need to be able to reach out to them when you need a shoulder to cry on, to brainstorm ideas for working out challenges, to solve day-to-day management problems, or to get a pat on the back when you hit your target goals.

For this reason, it's a good idea to continue to see a diabetes educator after you complete your initial training. Perhaps you come in once or twice a year with a list of questions because you want more information about a particular topic. Maybe your life situation has changed (thinking about pregnancy, going to college, retiring, or other life-changing events) or you are concerned that your diabetes has drifted out of control for a variety of reasons. Another way to stay connected with your diabetes educator is to attend a diabetes support group or an insulin pump support group that they facilitate. In this environment, you not only get support from your educators, but you get encouragement from others in the group—and you get to support others, too.

How Do You Keep on Keepin' On?

One of the most difficult parts of diabetes is staying motivated. There are daily tasks required to take good care of yourself—counting carbohydrates, checking blood glucose several times a day, making medication decisions, taking the medications, checking your feet, and on and on and on. All of these burdens can lead to a weariness that has been called "diabetes burnout." In order to avoid diabetes burnout, it's important to have a support team around you. And don't forget about the important role continual diabetes education plays in keeping you informed and motivated in your self-care.

So, find your coaches—your diabetes educators, doctors, friends and acquaintances who have diabetes, and family members. Utilize them as you continue to learn, solve problems, or deal with unusual situations. Let these people become members of your cheerleading squad.

Dr. Polonsky, author of *Diabetes Burnout,* concludes his book with this important message:

"The fundamental lesson to remember is that feeling stressed about living with diabetes is normal, feeling at war with diabetes is common, but problematic feelings like these can be conquered. With attention, kindness, and humor, you can overcome diabetes burnout and make peace with diabetes. This is not to suggest that you and diabetes will ever become the best of friends, but you can learn to make room for diabetes in your life. And, as you are certain to discover, this will actually improve the quality, and perhaps even quantity, of your life."

We feel that there is no more fitting message to end our book, too.

Meet Maddie

Maddie is a 71-year-old retired elementary school math teacher. She has had type 2 diabetes for about 16 years. She has taken pretty good care of her diabetes over the years, but her last two A1C readings were around 9%. She'd been taking two types of oral diabetes medications for years and had maxed out her doses on both. She also recently started blood pressure medication and found that she was spilling a small amount of protein in her urine. Maddie was concerned, frustrated, and feeling down. She felt she did a lot to manage her diabetes day to day, but she continued to have a number of high blood glucose levels each week.

Maddie's doctor told her that she really needed to think about starting insulin to control her blood glucose levels. She put her doctor off several times by bargaining for more time to "do better on her meal plan." One day, Maddie was reading the health section in the local paper and saw an announcement about a support group for people with diabetes who take insulin. She decided to attend the next group to get the lowdown on insulin from people who actually take it every day.

When Maddie introduced herself to the group, she let people know she didn't yet take insulin, but her doctor was recommending that she start. When the group ended, a woman came over to talk with her. She said that she had been in a similar situation about six months ago but finally bit the bullet and started taking a type of insulin at night. Then, because that wasn't enough to control her blood glucose levels, she started taking rapid-acting insulin before each of her meals. She said she had been amazed at how easy it was to give herself insulin, how much better she now felt, and how much more in control her blood glucose levels were. The woman also noted that her A1C had gone from 9.3 to 8.2% in six months. This woman suggested Maddie go see the dietitian at the local hospital's diabetes education program. She said that in three sessions, the dietitian taught her to do advanced carb counting, and now she was able to adjust her mealtime rapid-acting insulin dose based on her blood glucose levels and the amount of carbohydrate she planned to eat. The woman noted that she ended up paying for the sessions herself because her health plan would not, but she added it was not that expensive and was well worth it.

Maddie felt she had found a new friend—someone who understood her situation. She vowed to come back to the group's next meeting. She also promised herself she would call her doctor the next day to let her know she was ready to go on insulin and call the dietitian to schedule an appointment. Maddie was feeling a bit more positive about her ability and options to get her blood glucose under control.

Appendix 1

◆◆◆◆◆◆◆◆◆◆◆◆◆◆◆◆◆◆◆◆◆◆◆◆◆◆◆◆◆◆

Carb Counts of Everyday Foods

Starches

Includes breads, cereals, grains, starchy vegetables, crackers, snacks, beans, peas, lentils, and starchy foods prepared with fat.

Starches	Serving	Calories	Carb (g)	Fiber (g)
Breads				
Bagel	1/4 large	78	15	1
Bread, pumpernickel	1 slice	80	15	2
Bread, raisin	1 slice	71	14	1
Bread, rye	1 slice	83	16	2
Bread, white, reduced-calorie	2 slices	95	20	5
Bread, white	1 slice	67	12	1
Bread, whole-wheat	1 slice	69	13	2
English muffin	1/2	67	13	1
Hamburger bun or roll	1/2 small	60	11	1
Hot dog bun	1/2	61	11	1
Pita bread (6" dia.)	1/2	82	17	1
Roll, plain dinner	1 oz	85	14	1
Tortilla, corn, 6–7"	1	52	11	2
Tortilla, flour, 6"	1	112	15	1
Waffle, toaster-style, 4" square	1	96	15	1

Starches	Serving	Calories	Carb (g)	Fiber (g)
Cereals				
All-Bran	1/2 cup	81	23	10
Cheerios	2/3 cup	83	17	2
Corn flakes	2/3 cup	76	18	1
Cream of rice	3/4 cup	95	21	0
Cream of wheat	3/4 cup	98	21	1
Fiber One Bran Cereal	1/2 cup	59	24	14
Granola	1/4 cup	125	19	1
Granola cereal, low-fat	1/4 cup	86	18	1
Grits	1/2 cup	71	16	0
Kix	1 1/4 cups	110	25	3
Oatmeal, cooked	1/2 cup	73	13	2
Product 19	1 cup	100	25	1
Puffed rice	1 1/2 cups	80	19	0
Puffed wheat	1 1/2 cups	66	14	2
Raisin bran	1/2 cup	95	23	4
Rice Krispies	3/4 cup	77	17	0
Shredded wheat, plain	1/2 cup	83	20	3
Wheaties	3/4 cup	80	18	2
Crackers and Snacks				
Animal crackers	8	89	15	0
Crispbread	2 slices	73	16	3
Graham crackers	3	99	18	1
Matzos	3/4 oz	83	18	1
Melba toast	4 slices	78	15	1
Oyster crackers	20	86	14	1
Pita chips, baked	3/4 oz	86	12	0
Popcorn, microwave, 94% fat free	3 cups	65	14	3
Popcorn, microwave, with butter	3 cups	96	11	2
Popcorn, popped, no salt or fat added	3 cups	93	19	4
Potato chips	3/4 oz	114	11	1
Potato chips, baked	3/4 oz	82	17	2

Starches	Serving	Calories	Carb (g)	Fiber (g)
Pretzels, sticks/rings	3/4 oz	80	17	1
Rice cake, plain	2	70	15	1
Tortilla chips	3/4 oz	106	13	0
Tortilla chips, baked	3/4 oz	82	18	3
Grains				
Bulgur, cooked	1/2 cup	76	17	4
Cornmeal, dry, yellow	3 Tbsp	83	18	2
Couscous, cooked	1/3 cup	58	12	1
Flour, white	3 Tbsp	85	18	1
Kasha, cooked	1/2 cup	100	20	2
Millet, cooked	1/4 cup	52	10	1
Rice, white, long-grain, cooked	1/3 cup	68	15	0
Rice, brown, cooked	1/3 cup	71	15	1
Wheat germ, toasted	3 Tbsp	81	11	3
Pasta				
Macaroni, elbows, cooked	1/2 cup	111	22	1
Noodles, enriched egg, cooked	1/2 cup	110	20	1
Spaghetti, cooked	1/2 cup	91	18	1
Dried Beans, Peas, Lentils				
Beans, baked	1/3 cup	79	18	3
Beans, kidney, canned	1/2 cup	105	19	6
Beans, kidney, cooked	1/2 cup	112	20	6
Beans, lima, canned, drained	1/2 cup	99	18	6
Beans, lima, frozen, cooked	1/2 cup	76	14	4
Beans, navy, cooked	1/2 cup	129	24	6
Beans, pinto, cooked	1/2 cup	122	22	8
Beans, white, cooked	1/2 cup	125	23	6
Chickpeas, cooked	1/2 cup	134	23	6
Lentils, cooked	1/2 cup	115	20	8
Peas, split, cooked	1/2 cup	116	21	8
Peas, black-eyed, cooked	1/2 cup	100	17	6

Starches	Serving	Calories	Carb (g)	Fiber (g)
Starchy Vegetables				
Corn, canned, drained	1/2 cup	66	15	2
Corn, frozen, cooked	1/2 cup	66	16	2
Corn on cob, cooked,	1/2 large ear	66	16	2
Peas, green, canned, drained, no salt added	1 cup	39	8	4
Peas, green, frozen, cooked	1/2 cup	62	11	4
Plantain, ripe, cooked	1/3 cup, slices	59	16	1
Potato, baked with skin	3 oz	79	18	2
Potato, fresh, mashed (made with milk)	1/2 cup	85	19	2
Potato, white, peeled, boiled	3 oz	73	17	2
Squash, winter	1 cup	79	17	4
Vegetables, mixed, frozen, cooked (corn, peas, carrots)	1 cup	80	18	4
Vegetables, mixed, frozen, cooked (with pasta)	1 cup	80	15	5
Yams, cooked	1/2 cup	79	19	3

Vegetables

Includes raw, fresh, and canned vegetables and vegetable juices.

Vegetables	Serving	Calories	Carb (g)	Fiber (g)
Artichoke, cooked	1/2	30	7	1
Artichoke hearts, canned, drained	1	15	3	1
Asparagus, frozen, cooked	1/2 cup	25	4	1
Bean sprouts, fresh, cooked	1/2 cup	13	3	1
Beans (green, wax), canned, drained	1/2 cup	14	3	1
Beans, green, fresh, cooked	1/2 cup	22	5	2
Beets, canned, drained	1/2 cup	26	6	1

Vegetables	Serving	Calories	Carb (g)	Fiber (g)
Broccoli, fresh, cooked	1/2 cup	22	4	2
Brussels sprouts, frozen, cooked	1/2 cup	33	7	3
Cabbage, fresh, cooked	1/2 cup	17	3	2
Carrots, fresh, cooked	1/2 cup	35	8	3
Carrots, fresh, raw	1 cup	50	12	4
Cauliflower, fresh, raw	1 cup	25	5	3
Cauliflower, frozen, cooked	1/2 cup	17	3	2
Celery, fresh, raw	1 cup	17	4	2
Chard, Swiss, cooked	1/2 cup	18	4	2
Coleslaw mix	1 cup	17	3	2
Collard greens, fresh, cooked	1/2 cup	26	6	3
Cucumber, raw	1 cup	16	4	1
Eggplant, fresh, cooked	1/2 cup	17	4	1
Endive/escarole, raw	1 cup	9	2	2
Green (spring) onions	1 cup	32	7	3
Kale	1/2 cup	18	4	1
Kohlrabi, fresh, cooked	1/2 cup	24	6	1
Leeks, fresh, cooked	1/2 cup	16	4	1
Mixed vegetables (no corn, peas, pasta)	1/2 cup	20	3	1
Mushrooms, fresh, raw	1 cup	15	2	1
Mustard greens, fresh, cooked	1/2 cup	10	2	1
Okra, frozen, cooked	1/2 cup	34	5	3
Onions, fresh	1 cup	67	16	2
Onions, fresh, cooked	1/2 cup	46	11	2
Pea pods (snow peas), fresh, cooked	1/2 cup	34	6	2
Peas, sugar snap, frozen, uncooked	1/2 cup	30	5	2
Pepper, green bell, raw	1 cup, slices	18	4	2
Pepper, red bell, fresh, cooked	1/2 cup	19	5	1
Pepper, hot chili, green, canned	1/2 cup	25	3	3
Radishes	1 cup	20	4	2

Vegetables	Serving	Calories	Carb (g)	Fiber (g)
Sauerkraut, canned, rinsed, drained	1/2 cup	23	5	3
Spinach, canned, drained	1/2 cup	25	4	3
Spinach, fresh	1 cup	7	1	1
Squash, summer, fresh, cooked	1/2 cup	18	4	1
Squash, summer, raw	1 cup	18	4	1
Tomato juice	1/2 cup	21	5	1
Tomato sauce	1/2 cup	37	9	2
Tomatoes, canned, regular	1/2 cup	24	6	1
Tomatoes, raw	1 cup	32	7	2
Turnip greens, fresh, cooked	1/2 cup	14	3	3
Turnips, cooked, cubed	1/2 cup	17	4	2
Vegetable juice	1/2 cup	25	6	1
Water chestnuts, canned, drained	1/2 cup	40	9	3
Zucchini, fresh, cooked	1/2 cup, slices	14	4	1
Zucchini, raw	1 cup	18	4	1

Fruit

Includes fresh, dried, canned, and frozen fruit. Fruit juices are under nonalcoholic beverages.

Fruit	Serving	Calories	Carb (g)	Fiber (g)
Fruit, Fresh				
Apple, with peel, small	1 (4 oz)	54	14	3
Apricots	4	67	16	3
Banana, small	1 (6 inches)	72	19	2
Blackberries	3/4 cup	56	14	6
Blueberries	3/4 cup	62	16	3
Cantaloupe	1 cup	56	13	1
Cherries, sweet	12 (3 oz)	59	14	2
Figs, medium	2	74	19	3
Grapefruit	1/2	53	13	2

Fruit	Serving	Calories	Carb (g)	Fiber (g)
Grapes, seedless	17	60	15	1
Honeydew melon	1 cup	61	16	1
Kiwi	1	56	13	3
Mango	1/2 small	68	18	2
Nectarine	1 small	60	14	2
Orange	1 (6 1/2 oz)	62	15	3
Papaya	1 cup	55	14	3
Peach, medium	1 (6 oz)	57	14	2
Pear, large	1/2 (4 oz)	61	16	3
Pineapple	3/4 cup	56	15	2
Plums, small	2 (5 oz)	61	15	2
Raspberries, black, red	1 cup	60	14	8
Strawberries	1 1/4 cups	57	13	4
Tangerine, small	2 (8 oz)	81	20	3
Watermelon, cubed	1 1/4 cups	57	14	1
Fruit, Canned or Jarred, with Some Juice				
Applesauce, unsweetened	1/2 cup	52	14	2
Apricots, juice pack	1/2 cup	59	15	2
Cherries, sweet, juice pack	1/2 cup	68	17	2
Fruit cocktail, juice pack	1/2 cup	60	14	1
Grapefruit sections	3/4 cup	69	17	1
Mandarin oranges, juice pack	3/4 cup	69	18	1
Peaches, juice pack	1/2 cup	55	14	2
Pears, juice pack	1/2 cup	62	16	2
Pineapple, juice pack	1/2 cup	74	20	1
Plums, juice pack	1/2 cup	73	19	1
Fruit, Dried				
Apples, rings	4	63	17	2
Apricots, halves	8	67	18	2
Dates	3	69	19	2
Figs	1 1/2	71	18	3
Raisins, dark, seedless	2 Tbsp	54	14	1

Milk and Yogurt

Includes dairy-like foods.

Milks and milk products	Total Serving	Calories	Carb (g)	Fat (g)	Protein (g)
Nonfat or Low-Fat					
Acidophilus milk, fat-free	1 cup	128	11	5	8
Buttermilk, fat-free	1 cup	98	12	0	8
Buttermilk, low-fat	1 cup	99	12	2	8
Lactaid, fat-free	1 cup	80	13	0	8
Milk, 1%	1 cup	110	13	3	8
Milk, 2%	1 cup	130	12	5	8
Milk, evaporated, fat-free	1/2 cup	100	15	0	10
Milk, fat-free	1 cup	90	13	0	10
Yogurt, flavored, fat-free, sweetened with Splenda	6 oz	80	11	0	7
Yogurt, nonfat, plain	6 oz	82	12	0	8
Yogurt, plain, low-fat	6 oz	107	12	3	9
Whole Milks					
Milk, evaporated, whole	1/2 cup	169	13	10	9
Milk, goat, whole	1 cup	168	11	10	9
Milk, whole	1 cup	150	12	8	8
Yogurt, plain, made from whole milk	1 cup	160	12	8	9
Dairy-Like Foods					
Chocolate milk, fat-free	1 cup	160	31	0	9
Chocolate milk, whole	1 cup	208	26	9	8
Eggnog, whole milk	1/2 cup	171	17	10	5
Rice drink, fat-free or 1%, plain	1 cup	90	18	2	1
Rice drink, low-fat, flavored	1 cup	122	25	2	1
Soy milk, light	1 cup	100	15	2	5
Soy milk, regular, plain	1 cup	115	11	4	8
Yogurt, low-carb, sweetened with Splenda	6 oz	70	5	3	5
Yogurt with fruit, low-fat	6 oz	150	28	2	6

Meat and Other Foods That Contain Mostly Protein and Fat

Most meats (such as beef, poultry, seafood, and eggs) contain no carbohydrate. However, some foods in this food group—processed meats, tofu, cheeses, and peanut butter—contain very small amounts of carbohydrate.

	Total Serving	Calories	Carb (g)	Fat (g)
Beef, jerky, dried	1 oz	116	3	7
Beef sticks, smoked	1 oz	156	2	14
Cheese, American, fat-free	1 slice	31	3	0
Cheese, American, regular	1 slice	79	0	7
Cheese, cheddar, regular	1 slice	113	0	9
Cheese, Monterey jack, regular	1 slice	110	0	9
Cheese, Swiss, regular	1 slice	106	2	8
Cottage cheese, low-fat (1%)	1/4 cup	41	2	1
Cottage cheese, fat-free	1/4 cup	40	3	0
Fish sticks	2	139	12	7
Peanut butter, chunky	1 Tbsp	94	4	8
Peanut butter, smooth	1 Tbsp	94	3	8
Ricotta, part-skim	1/4 cup	86	3	5
Tempeh	1/4 cup	80	4	5
Tofu	1/2 cup	183	5	11

Sweets and Sugary Foods

The grams of carbohydrate per serving in this group vary quite a bit. The fat and calorie content vary quite a bit too.

Sweets	Serving	Calories	Carb (g)	Fat (g)
Angel food cake, not frosted	1 slice (2 oz)	128	29	0
Brownie, unfrosted	2" square	115	18	5
Cake, frosted	2" square	175	29	6

Sweets	Serving	Calories	Carb (g)	Fat (g)
Cake, unfrosted	2" square	97	17	3
Cookies, chocolate chip	2 medium	156	19	9
Cookies, gingersnap, regular	3	87	16	2
Cookies, sandwich, cream filling	2 small	93	14	4
Cookies, sugar-free	3 small	141	20	7
Cookies, vanilla wafers	5	88	15	3
Cupcake, frosted, small	1	174	29	6
Danish pastry, fruit type (4 1/4" dia.)	1 pastry	263	34	13
Donut, plain cake	1 medium	196	21	11
Donut, glazed (3 3/4" dia.)	1	239	30	12
Fruit spreads, 100% fruit	1 1/2 Tbsp	60	15	0
Granola bar	1	134	18	6
Granola bar, chewy, low-fat	1	109	22	2
Honey	1 Tbsp	64	17	0
Ice cream	1/2 cup	165	15	10
Ice cream, fat-free	1/2 cup	90	22	0
Ice cream, light	1/2 cup	120	16	5
Ice cream, no sugar added	1/2 cup	115	15	6
Jam or preserves, regular	1 Tbsp	48	13	0
Jelly, regular	1 Tbsp	52	13	0
Pie, fruit, 2 crust	1/6 pie	284	42	13
Pie, pumpkin or custard	1/8 pie	168	22	8
Pudding, regular, reduced-fat milk	1/2 cup	141	26	2
Pudding, sugar-free, fat-free, fat-free milk	1/2 cup	70	12	0
Sherbet	1/2 cup	138	29	2
Sorbet	1/2 cup	130	31	0
Sweet roll	1	264	36	12
Syrup, pancake, light	2 Tbsp	50	13	0
Syrup, pancake, regular	1 Tbsp	50	13	0
Yogurt, frozen, fat-free	1/3 cup	66	13	0
Yogurt, frozen, regular	1/2 cup	110	19	3

Fats

Many of the foods in this group—margarine, butter, oils, olives, bacon, and sausage—contain no carbohydrate. Several foods in this food group—nuts, salad dressings, low-fat and fat-free mayonnaise, and spreads—contain very small amounts of carbohydrate.

	Total Serving	Calories	Carb (g)	Fat (g)
Nuts				
Almonds, raw	1 oz	164	6	14
Cashews, raw	1 oz	157	9	12
Peanuts, raw	1 oz	161	5	14
Pecans, raw	1 oz	196	4	20
Pumpkin seeds, roasted, no salt added	1 oz	148	4	12
Walnuts	1 oz	183	4	18
Salad Dressings, Spreads, Etc.				
Hummus	1 Tbsp	23	2	1
Ketchup	1 Tbsp	15	4	0
Mayonnaise, regular	1 Tbsp	57	4	5
Mayonnaise, fat-free	1 Tbsp	13	3	0
Mayonnaise, reduced-fat	1 Tbsp	49	1	5
Mustard, yellow	1 Tbsp	10	1	1
Salad dressing, blue cheese	1 Tbsp	76	1	8
Salad dressing, blue cheese, reduced-fat	1 Tbsp	14	2	0
Salad dressing, Caesar	1 Tbsp	78	1	9
Salad dressing, Caesar, reduced-fat	1 Tbsp	17	3	1
Salad dressing, French	1 Tbsp	73	3	7
Salad dressing, French, fat-free	1 Tbsp	21	5	0
Salad dressing, French, reduced-fat	1 Tbsp	37	5	2
Salad dressing, Italian	1 Tbsp	43	2	4
Salad dressing, Italian, fat-free	1 Tbsp	7	1	0

	Total Serving	Calories	Carb (g)	Fat (g)
Salad dressing, Italian, reduced-fat	1 Tbsp	11	1	1
Salad dressing, Ranch	1 Tbsp	73	1	8
Salad dressing, Ranch, fat-free	1 Tbsp	17	4	0
Salad dressing, Ranch, reduced-fat	1 Tbsp	33	2	3
Salad dressing, Thousand Island	1 Tbsp	59	3	6
Salad dressing, Thousand Island, fat-free	1 Tbsp	21	5	0
Salad dressing, Thousand Island, reduced-fat	1 Tbsp	31	3	2

Beverages: Nonalcoholic

Many drinks don't contain carbohydrate, but some do. This list covers fruit juices and other drinks (except milk).

Beverage	Serving	Calories	Carb (g)
Apple juice/cider	1/2 cup	58	15
Caffe latte, nonfat milk	8 oz	67	10
Caffe latte, whole mile	8 oz	136	11
Caffe mocha, nonfat milk, no whipped cream	8 oz	112	21
Caffe mocha, 2% milk, no whipped cream	8 oz	136	21
Coffee, black	1 cup	2	0
Coffee, with 2 Tbsp half & half	1 cup	41	1
Fruit juice blends, 100% juice	1/3 cup	50	12
Grape juice	1/3 cup	50	13
Orange juice, fresh	1/2 cup	56	13
Pineapple juice, canned	1/2 cup	70	17
Prune juice	1/3 cup	59	15
Soda, cola	12 oz	131	34
Soda, cola, diet	12 oz	7	1
Soda, ginger ale	12 oz	124	32

Beverage	Serving	Calories	Carb (g)
Soda, lemon lime	12 oz	139	35
Sport drink, regular	16 oz	112	28
Sport drink, sweetened with a no-calorie sweetener	16 oz	20	4

Beverages: Alcoholic

Most of the calories in alcoholic beverages are provided by the alcohol. Most alcoholic beverages contain no carbohydrate, but other beverages do, so consider that when you order mixed drinks. When you drink alcohol, be careful because alcohol can either make your blood glucose rise or fall too low. See pages 46–47 for more information on the use of alcoholic beverages. Note that these are average figures. Different products may have different nutritional value.

Beverage	Serving	Carb (g)
Beer, regular	12 oz	13
Beer, light	12 oz	5
Brandy	1 1/2 oz (1 shot)	0
Liquor, any type (e.g., gin, rum, vodka)	1 1/2 oz (1 shot)	0
Liqueur, any type (e.g., Kahlua, crème de menthe)	1 1/2 oz (1 shot)	14–18
Wine, red	4 oz	3
Wine, white	4 oz	1

Appendix 2

◆◆◆◆◆◆◆◆◆◆◆◆◆◆◆◆◆◆◆◆◆◆◆◆◆◆◆

Carb Counting Resources

Basic Resources

If you're counting carbs, you'll need resources for three categories of foods.

1. Foods with a Nutrition Facts label
2. Foods without a Nutrition Facts label (e.g., fresh produce)
3. Restaurant foods

1. FOODS WITH A NUTRITION FACTS LABEL

If available, this is the best resource you have. For many products, the Nutrition Facts label is readily available, and it's the most accurate and up to date, and the least expensive, source of carbohydrate information. Use the **Total Carbohydrate** grams. There is no need to pay attention to or count the **grams of Sugars**. These are already factored into the grams of carbohydrate. If the fiber count is higher than 5 grams per serving (meal or snack), consider subtracting half the grams of fiber from the total carbohydrate count of the food or foods in a meal or snack.

2. FOODS WITHOUT A NUTRITION FACTS LABEL

This applies to foods such as fresh fruit, vegetables, and starchy vegetables, which you purchase in the produce area of the grocery store. For foods like these, a book, online database, or carbohydrate counting app is usually your best resource.

- *The Diabetes Carbohydrate and Fat Gram Guide*, by Lea Ann Holzmeister, RD, CDE (American Diabetes Association, 4th edition, 2010, 730 pages). This book provides the carbohydrate count, as well as other nutrition information, for thousands of foods, including fruits, vegetables, and other produce; meats, poultry, and seafood; desserts; many foods you know by brand name; frozen entrées; and more.

- *The CalorieKing Calorie, Fat & Carbohydrate Counter*, by Allan Borushek (Family Health Publications, 2010, 304 pages). This book provides the calorie, fat, and carbohydrate information for thousands of basic and brand names foods.

- *Barbara Kraus' Calories and Carbohydrates*, by Barbara Kraus (Signet, 16th edition, 2005, 500 pages). This book provides the carbohydrate and calorie count for more than 8,000 foods, including fruits, vegetables, and other produce; meats, poultry, and seafood; desserts; many foods you know by brand name; frozen entrées; and more.

- *The Complete Book of Food Counts*, by Corinne T. Netzer (Dell, 8th edition, 2008, 900 pages). This book provides the carbohydrate count for thousands of foods, including fruits, vegetables, and other produce; meats, poultry, and seafood; desserts; many foods you know by brand name; frozen entrées; and more.

- See online resources on page 149.

3. RESTAURANT FOODS

When you're eating out, it's tougher to get the nutrition information for the foods you choose. These resources may help.

- Chain restaurants' websites. The websites for many chain restaurants provide nutrition information, including information about carbohydrates. In addition, numerous third-party websites provide nutrition information for restaurants.

- *American Diabetes Association Guide to Healthy Restaurant Eating*, by Hope Warshaw, MMSc, RD, CDE, BC, ADM (American Diabetes Association, 4th edition, 2009, 800 pages). This guide provides the basics about diabetes nutrition and meal planning goals, strategies for healthy restaurant eating, and information on how to best estimate restaurant portions. Included is nutrition information for 5,000 menu items from more than 60 major restaurant chains.

- *Eat Out, Eat Right,* by Hope Warshaw, MMSc, RD, CDE (Surrey Books, 2008, 3rd edition, 300 pages). This easy-to-carry guide provides practical and realistic solutions to eating healthier when eating out in nearly every type of restaurant—from fast food to fine dining—and nearly every cuisine—from Italian and Mexican to Indian and Japanese.

- *Nutrition in the Fast Lane—The Fast Food Dining Guide* (Franklin Publishing Inc., Indianapolis, IN). To order this booklet, call 800-634-1993 or go to **www.fastfoodfacts.com**. This booklet, updated annually, provides the nutrition information for 54 of the country's most popular chain restaurants.

Helpful Software and Websites

Some software allows you to track nutrient intake. Some websites provide an option to download data to a home PC, PDA, iPod, or other device. The website **www.diabetesnet.com** provides an excellent listing of blood glucose monitoring software and online resources.

- **www.ars.usda.gov/nutrientdata**. This is the USDA's National Nutrient Database for Standard Reference. This database, updated annually, contains extensive nutrition information for about 8,000 commonly eaten foods. It is downloadable to a PC and searchable, downloadable to a PDA, or searchable online. This database is in the public domain, so there's no cost to download it or use it online. (This database forms the core of many of the commercial nutrient count books and websites.)

- **www.mypyramidtracker.gov**. This government online dietary assessment, part of the MyPyramid website, provides information on diet quality, related nutrition messages, and links to nutrient information. After providing a day's worth of dietary information, an overall evaluation comparing the amounts of food you ate to current nutritional guidance is provided.

- **www.healthydiningfinder.com**. This website allows you to search for restaurants that offer a selection of healthier menu items and view the nutrition information for those items. You can search by zip code and/or other criteria. The site was developed with a grant from the Centers for Disease Control and Prevention (CDC) and in collaboration with the National Restaurant Association. New restaurants are added regularly.

Additional websites for nutrition information:
  - **www.calorieking.com**
  - **www.myfooddiary.com**
  - **www.nutritiondata.com**
  - **www.dietfacts.com**
  - **www.chowbaby.com/fastfood/fast_food_nutrition.asp**

Note: look for iPhone, iPad, iPod, Blackberry, and Android apps.

FURTHER ONLINE SOFTWARE AND WEBSITE RESOURCES

The following websites provide software or services that offer one or more of the following:
  ▎ carbohydrate counts of foods and ability to track intake
  ▎ ability to track blood glucose results by downloading to your meter
  ▎ integration and analysis of data
  ▎ ability to communicate about the data online with a health care provider

  - **www.dia-log.com**
  - **www.diabetespilot.com**
  - **www.healthengage.com**
  - **www.logforlife.com**
  - **www.sugarstats.com**
  - **www.glucosebuddy.com**

Carb "Guesstimating" Equipment

Learn how much food equals certain amounts of carbohydrate by using measuring equipment. Initially, use this equipment regularly. As your skills improve, your skilled (and honest) eyes will serve you well both at home and when you eat at restaurants. Weigh and measure your foods weekly or more often to make sure your eyes (and portions) have not grown with time. The more you use these tools, the more precise your carb counts and amounts of foods will be.

Consider these carb guesstimating tools:

- Set of measuring cups from 1/4 cup to 1 cup
- Set of measuring spoons from 1/4 teaspoon to 1 tablespoon
- Food scale: you can purchase an inexpensive food scale for between $5 and $15. Use this to measure meats, fruits, breads, and other foods that don't come with a Nutrition Facts label on the packaging.

    There are more expensive food scales ($40–$100) that have more advanced features, such as providing the gram weight of foods and grams of carbohydrate based on an internal database.

There are also specialized items out there to help you visualize serving sizes. Try searching for "portion control products" on the Internet.

Appendix 3

Record-Keeping Forms

Carb Counting and Blood Glucose Results Record

Day/Date:_____

| Time/meal | Diabetes medicines | | Food | | Carb grams |
	Type	Amount	Type	Amount	

Notes about day:

Blood glucose results							
Fasting/ before b'fast/ time	After b'fast/ time	Before lunch/ time	After lunch/ time	Before dinner/ time	After dinner/ time	Before bed/ time	Other/ time

Carb Counting and Blood Glucose Results Record

Day/Date: <u>Tuesday, June 3</u>

Time/meal	Diabetes medicines		Food		Carb grams
	Type	Amount	Type	Amount	
6:45 a/ breakfast	Lispro	4 units	Shredded Wheat 'n Bran with Cheerios Milk Banana	1/2 cup 3/4 cup 1 cup 1 large	
12:30p	Lispro	5 units	Sub sandwich– 12" turkey, ham, cheese, lettuce, tomato, onions, pickles, mustard Pretzels	1 2 1/2 oz bag	
5:00 p			Apple	1 large	
7:15 p/ dinner	Lispro	7 units			
10:00 p	Glargine	14 units			

Notes about day:
Went for a walk after dinner. Felt a bit low an hour after return (see other BG).

Blood glucose results							
Fasting/ before b'fast/ time	After b'fast/ time	Before lunch/ time	After lunch/ time	Before dinner/ time	After dinner/ time	Before bed/ time	Other/ time
92/ 6:30 a	179/ 9:10 a						
		123/ 12:30 p	89/ 2:00 p				

Build Your Food and Carb Counting Database

As you begin to use carb counting to control your diabetes, you will find out the carb count of many foods—the crackers you buy, the apples you usually choose, your favorite ice cream, frozen entrée, or restaurant meal. Rather than having to keep a mental list of the carb counts of these foods or having to look them up every time, start to build your Carb Count Database. This information helps you keep track of the foods, the servings you usually eat, the carb count, and any notes you want to record. For example, maybe you find that a particular food does (or does not) make your blood glucose rise as much as you thought it would or a particular food is a good snack before exercise or on a full day of hiking.

You can keep this record in a notebook, a computer file, or on a handheld device. Keep it in a convenient place and in a format that works for you.

CARB COUNT DATABASE

Meal	Amount I Eat	Carb Count (grams)	Notes (effect on blood glucose level, what you would do next time you eat this, etc.)

SAMPLE CARB COUNT DATABASE

Meal	Amount I Eat	Carb Count (grams)	Notes (effect on blood glucose level, what you would do next time you eat this, etc.)
Bagel (Dunkin' Donuts)—pumpernickel	1	70	More carbs than I thought!
Grandma Grace's Apple Cobbler	3/4 cup	35 (from recipe analysis)	Don't need as much insulin as I thought I would to cover it.
Domino's cheese pizza with onions and mushrooms—hand-tossed	2 slices of 14" pizza	45	Raises my blood glucose most 3 hours after I eat it.
Healthy Choice Ginger Chicken Hunan	1 entrée	59	Quick rise in blood glucose
Weight Watcher's Garden Lasagna	1 entrée	30	Works well.

Here's another example of a chart you can use for your database of foods.

PERSONAL FOOD DATABASE

Food	Amount I Eat	Carb Count (grams)	Notes (effect on blood glucose level, what you would do next time you eat this, etc.)

SAMPLE PERSONAL FOOD DATABASE

Food	Amount I Eat	Carb Count (grams)	Notes (effect on blood glucose level, what you would do next time you eat this, etc.)
Dry cereal, Shredded Wheat 'n Bran mixed with Raisin Bran	1 cup (1/2 cup of each)	59	1 hour after eating—BG 185 Decrease amount of cereal or take more rapid-acting insulin
McDonald's Quarter Pounder with small fries and 1% milk	1 1 1	37 26 13 76	2 hours after eating—BG 165 Took 5 units of rapid-acting insulin to cover meal— worked well

Index

Other Titles from the American Diabetes Association

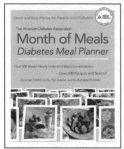

American Diabetes Association
Month of Meals Diabetes Meal Planner
by American Diabetes Association
The bestselling Month of Meals™ series is all here—newly updated and collected into one complete, authoritative volume! Forget about the hassle of planning meals and spending hours making menus fit your diabetes management. With this invaluable guide, you'll have millions of daily menu combinations at your fingertips. Simply pick a menu for each meal, prepare your recipes, and enjoy a full day of delicious meals tailored specifically to you. It's as easy as that!
Order no. 4679-01; Price $22.95

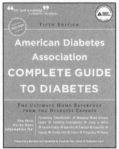

American Diabetes Association
Complete Guide to Diabetes, 5th Edition
by American Diabetes Association
When it comes to managing diabetes, knowledge is your most powerful tool. From describing the different types of diabetes to breaking down the details of blood glucose monitoring, the *Complete Guide to Diabetes* covers everything a person with diabetes needs to know to stay healthy and in control. Completely revised to contain the latest information on research, medications, and treatments, this book has the answer to any question you may have about diabetes.
Order no. 4809-05; Price $22.95

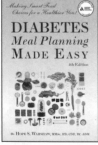

Diabetes Meal Planning Made Easy, 4th Edition
by Hope S. Warshaw, MMSc, RD, CDE, BC-ADM
This new edition of the meal-planning bestseller uncovers the secrets to healthy eating with diabetes—from the basics of what to eat to the practical skills of shopping, planning nutritious meals, and even eating healthy restaurant meals. You don't have to change your life to eat healthy, but you might be surprised to learn how eating healthy can change your life!
Order no. 4706-04; Price $16.95

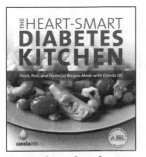

The Heart-Smart Diabetes Kitchen: Fresh, Fast, and Flavorful Recipes Made with Canola Oil

by the American Diabetes Association and CanolaInfo

Bring the taste of fresh, natural ingredients and wholesome meals to your table. Featuring over 150 recipes made with canola oil, this cookbook allows you to serve dishes that are low in saturated fat and cholesterol but high in flavor in no time. It's just what the doctor, and your inner chef, ordered,

Order no. 4677-01; Price $18.95

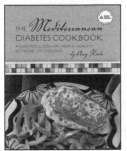

The Mediterranean Diabetes Cookbook

by Amy Riolo

Mediterranean cuisine uses healthful, fresh ingredients, and when it is paired with the moderate Mediterranean lifestyle, you can enjoy delicious, traditional, and naturally diabetes-friendly dishes. Award-winning food writer Amy Riolo introduces you to a new world of health, well-being, and flavor. Leave behind tired, watered-down diabetes recipes and regain the joys of eating.

Order no. 4674-01; $19.95

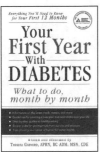

Your First Year with Diabetes

by Theresa Garnero, CDE, APRN, BC-ADM, MSN

Diabetes happens. It can happen to anyone—*even you*. If diabetes has left you feeling confused or angry, then it's time to turn to Theresa Garnero. Straightforward and easy to read, *Your First Year with Diabetes* will help you manage and deal with your diabetes—day to day, week to week, and month to month. You'll learn about medication, exercise, meal planning, and lifestyle and emotional issues at a pace that suits you.

Order no. 5024-01; Price $16.95

To order these and other great American Diabetes Association titles, call **1-800-232-6733** or visit **www.shopdiabetes.org**.
American Diabetes Association titles are also available in bookstores nationwide.